Sex Lover's Book of Lists

Ron Louis
David Copeland

REWARD

Library of Congress Cataloging-in-Publication Data

Louis, Ron.
    Sex lover's book of lists / Ron Louis and David Copeland.
      p. cm.
    ISBN 0-7352-0216-8
    1. Sex—Miscellanea. 2. Sex customs—Miscellanea. 3. Lists.
I. Copeland, David. II. Title.

HQ23.L68 2001
306.7—dc21   00-045928

Printed in the United States of America

10 9 8 7 6 5 4 3 2 1

ISBN 0-7352-0216-8

REWARD BOOKS
Paramus, NJ 07652

This book is dedicated to all the people who have been persecuted because of their sexuality—people who have lost their jobs, been imprisoned, or even been killed for being forward-thinking or "off the grid" in their con-sensual sexual activity. Our hats are off to you—thanks for paving the way to the (admittedly spotty) level of sexual freedom we enjoy today.

ACKNOWLEDGMENTS

———◆———

We want to thank Jennifer Corbin and her staff at the Kinsey Institute for going out of their way to be helpful to us on this project. We'd also like to thank Gene Brissie, Tess Woods, and Reward Books, as well as Roan Kaufman and Dmitri Bilgere, without whom this book would have been impossible. We'd also like to thank Steve Earle, Robert Hatch, Cliff Barry, Tom Daly, Pete A., Murray K., Angel Boris, Tom Waits, Carolyn Songin, Jennifer Taylor, Heather Simmons, and *Fight Club*.

INTRODUCTION

———◆———

Thanks for buying *Sex Lover's Book of Lists*.

Creating this book has been a real learning experience. We've been amazed by what we've learned. This book has turned out to be three things: a history of sexual attitudes (which are stranger than you might think!), a resource list about sexuality, and a healthy dose of good old entertainment. We hope you will find it fun and informative.

In all of our work we deal with sex, at least on some level. In *How to Succeed with Women* we helped men learn how to develop relationships with women and get women into bed; in *How to Succeed with Men* we helped women learn the same things, as well as teaching them how to develop committed long-term relationships in which sexuality could remain alive and vital. In our dating and relationship coaching business and at our seminars we do the same things. In this book we continue our campaign to help people "open up" about sex. After reading this book and seeing all the trouble sexual repression and shame can cause, it may become easier for you to give up some of your sexual "hang-ups" and to enjoy your life, and your sexuality, even more.

You can contact us at http://datingcoaches.com, http://howtosucceedwithwomen.com, or http://howtosucceedwithmen.com to send us any sex lists you may have, to look at lists other people have sent in, or find out about our dating coaching and seminars. You can also email us at succeed@pobox.com or write us at P.O. Box 55094, Madison, WI 53705.

Now have fun with *Sex Lover's Book of Lists!*

Ron Louis and David Copeland

CONTENTS

Contents

◆

Chapter 2 *Biology*   *57*

Contents

Chapter 3 *Sex Industry* **115**

Contents

◆

Chapter 4   Law   153

◆

Chapter 5   Internet   173

◆

Chapter 6   Other Cultures   183

Contents

Contents

CHAPTER 1

History
and Sex

Historic Medical Myths About Women's Sexuality (and a Couple About Men's)

We hear a lot these days about how little money goes to research women's illnesses. After reading this section, you may wish that women's illnesses had been of *less* interest to doctors in the past:

1. German-Swiss physician Philippus Paracelsus (1493–1541) spoke of an illness called "womb fury." "The womb changes into an unfavorable one, which . . . results in a contraction of the uterus and takes away all reason. If the womb neither feels, nor has the proper substance, then it is cold. This causes . . . a sharp acid in the uterus. The contraction . . . and spasm also force the other limbs into spasm and tetanus, for they become contaminated by the womb also . . . vapor and smoke come out of the womb to the organs around it." Thank heavens this terrible affliction has been cured by modern science!

2. The ancients believed that women's wombs moved throughout their bodies and could cause harm to other organs. This led to the ancient Egyptian treatment of burning bad-smelling substances near a woman's nose, in order to repel her uterus back to its proper place.

3. Many tribal cultures believed that a woman who is menstruating is medically unfit to take part in a sweat lodge.

4. In the 1800s, doctors believed that too much sex caused a woman to become frigid and would drive her to hysteria or insanity.

5. It used to be believed that cunnilingus causes cancer of the tongue.

2

6. Similarly, in the Middle Ages doctors believed that one drop of semen is formed from forty drops of blood. (Okay, this one is more about men, but it's still interesting).

7. It is still commonly believed as a medical fact that if a woman's hymen does not bleed on the wedding night, she is not a virgin. (There are a lot ways a woman can lose her hymen before having intercourse, including sports, masturbation, or insertion of fingers or other objects.)

8. It used to be commonly believed that intercourse during menstruation was harmful to either the woman, the man, or both.

9. Women have semen just like men, but if they went without sex for too long, the semen would accumulate and cause hysteria. This was promulgated by Galen (130–201 B.C.), a Greek physician.

10. Women's uteruses have seven chambers, three for male babies, three for female, and one for hermaphrodite babies. This idea was popular in the 1500s, and medical texts had drawings of these seven-chambered wombs.

11. Women who wanted education, didn't like keeping the house, or who generally gave any trouble to their husbands in any way were considered hysterical. *Hysteria* was believed to be a real medical condition all the way into the early twentieth century and was treated by sending the "hysterical" woman to an asylum. There the woman was often tied to a cot and dunked into freezing-cold water—basically a form of torture to impel her toward obedience. Hysterectomy was also a popular medical treatment for hysteria.

12. Many doctors believed that healthy women did not enjoy sex. If they did, they were hysterical or insane. Back to the ice-cold baths.

13. It was said that men have a limited, finite amount of semen, and too much sex with women uses it up, forever.

After all, the sexual life of adult women is a dark continent of psychology.

—Sigmund Freud

Historically Believed Effects of Masturbation

Speaking of deep thinking, an eighteenth-century Swiss physician named S.A.D. Tissot (1728–1797) came up with the idea that the body can "waste" its resources. This "wastage" was most debilitating when it came in the form of masturbation. Parents spent the next hundred and fifty years trying to prevent their children from masturbating. Thanks a lot, S.A.D.!

Here's what Tissot—and doctors for a hundred and fifty years after him—thought masturbation caused:

1. Acne
2. Backache
3. Blindness
4. Constipation
5. Death
6. Decay of bodily powers
7. Epilepsy
8. Gout
9. Infertility
10. Madness
11. Nymphomania
12. Use of profanity
13. Vomiting

We'll get to the historical cures for masturbation later. Meanwhile, it turns out that many of the symptoms attributed to masturbation were actually symptoms of untreated syphilis. How about that?

> *The good thing about masturbation is that you don't have to dress up for it.*
>
> —Truman Capote

———◆———

Sex Museums, Galleries, and Museums That Have Sexual Collections

1. *Bibliothèque Nationale, Paris.* Erotic Greek pottery, erotic prints, and literature.

2. *The British Library in the British Museum, Museum Street, London.* Has a huge collection of historic erotic arts.

3. *The Delta Collection of the Library of Congress, Washington, DC.* Large collection of old erotic materials sized by customs officials.

4. *The Edward Nikola Collection of Erotic Art, Vienna.* Includes works by Gustav Klimt and Egon Schiele.

5. *The Institute for the Advanced Study of Human Sexuality,* 11523 Frankin Street, San Francisco, CA 94109. (415) 928-1133.

6. *The Kinsey Institute for Sex Research, Bloomington, IN.* Along with books and magazines, they also have an extensive collection of erotic video, microfilmed arts, and a small gallery. The staff is friendly and quite helpful, though you have to have a legitimate reason to use their archives. The Kinsey

Institute, Morrison 313, Indiana University, Bloomington, IN 47405. (812)855-7686.

7. *The Leather Archives and Museum, Chicago, IL.* The Leather archives is dedicated to the history of the underground fetish world, and, unlike many of the collections on this list, is easily accessible and open to the public. 505 N. Clark St., Chicago, IL 60640. (312) 878-6360.

8. *The Vatican Library, Rome.* Speaking of not easily accessible, the Vatican Library's erotic collection is rumored to be one of the finest in the world. It is also sometimes said not even to exist. If your travel plans include Rome, they probably won't let you into it, but you can try.

9. *Erotic Art Gallery,* Drop in for a visit! 701 East Los Olas Blvd, Ft. Lauderdale, FL 33301. (305) 524-2100.

10. *Feitiço Erotic Art Gallery,* Go visit! 1821 West North Avenue, Chicago, IL 60622. (773)384-0586 http://www.feitico.com/

What is pornography to one man is the laughter of genius to another.

—D. H. Lawrence

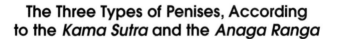

The Three Types of Penises, According to the *Kama Sutra* and the *Anaga Ranga*

You didn't think that a penis is a penis is a penis, did you? According to two ancient texts—the *Kama Sutra* and the *Anaga Ranga* (the essential guides to sexuality)—there are three types of penises. Also, it's not a penis, it's a *lingam*.

1. **The Hare.** Not longer than six finger-widths (about five inches) when erect. This man's semen is sweet.

2. **The Bull.** Not shockingly, this penis is larger than the hare. The Bull is not longer than nine finger-widths (about seven inches) when erect.

3. **The Horse.** About twelve finger-widths (around ten inches) in length. Puts the old song lyric, "There was an old woman who swallowed a horse" in a new, yet somewhat disgusting, light.

Beware of the man who denounces women writers; his penis is tiny and he cannot spell.

—Erica Jong

———◆———

The Three Types of Vaginas, According to the *Kama Sutra* and the *Anaga Ranga*

Not content in naming the three types of penises, these fine works went on to name the three types of vaginas. And by the way, it's not a vagina, it's a *yoni.* We're sorry if some of these vaginal classifications sound vaguely insulting. We're just reporting the historical facts here.

1. **The Deer.** The deer yoni is no deeper than six finger-widths, or about five inches. This deer is usually a small woman, as you can imagine.

2. **The Mare.** This yoni is no deeper than nine finger-widths, or about seven inches. This woman does not climax easily, and her fluids smell like a lotus. Fair enough.

3. **The Elephant.** About twelve finger-widths, or about ten inches deep. She is known for being of large dimension. How about that.

> *The evidence indicates that woman is, on the whole, biologically superior to man.*
>
> —Ashley Montagu

Rules from a Brothel, Dated 1347

Some things never change; some things do.

Rules from a 1347 Brothel:

1. Each Saturday the brothel keeper and the doctor shall examine all the girls at the brothel. Any girl who is ill shall be kept apart so that no young man may catch her disease.

2. If any girl gets pregnant, the keeper of the brothel shall make sure that the baby is not killed and shall arrange for the providing of the child.

3. The brothel keeper shall not allow any Jew to enter. If any Jew enters and has carnal knowledge of any girl, he shall be imprisoned and whipped.

> *You can lead a horticulture but you can't make her think.*
>
> —Dorothy Parker

Ben Franklin's Reasons for a Young Man to Date an Older Woman

Ben had ideas about everything.

1. They have more life experience, and so "their conversation is more improving, and more lastingly agreeable."

2. Older women are easier to get along with, because "when women cease to be handsome they study to be good."

3. They won't have children, attending "much inconvenience." Franklin knew about this himself, having had a child out of wedlock before his marriage and, in his youth, being much prone toward assignations with "low women who would fall my way."

4. They can keep quiet about things, and can conduct an affair without getting caught. Also, if people do find out about such an affair, it's better than if you were seeing a prostitute.

5. They've had more practice at sex, so are better at it.

6. Because if you "debauch a virgin" you can ruin her life—but the sin is less with an older woman.

7. While you might make a young woman miserable, you are more likely to make an older woman happy.

8. And lastly—they are so grateful.

A soldier's discharged and he may be bald and toothless yet he'll find a pretty young woman to go to bed with. But a woman! Her beauty is gone with the first gray hair. She can spend her time consulting the oracles and fortune-tellers, but they'll never send her a husband.

—Aristophanes

Famous Historic Sex Prudes

These people had more of an effect on your life than you think. Are you circumcised? Sir Johnathan Hutchinson may have had something to do with it. Ever eat a Graham cracker, or corn flakes? Both of these foods were designed with stopping masturbation in mind. Ever feel a vague sense of shame about masturbating, sexuality, or your fantasies? Thank any of these yo-yos for that.

1. Simon André Tissot (1728–1797). A Swiss physician, his book, *A Treatise on the Diseases Produced by Onanism* was published in France in 1741 and translated into English in 1832, and popular all the while in between. Tissot was one of the first, if not *the* first, doctor to attack masturbation (or *onanism,* as it was also called) as the root cause of just about every physical ill.

Tissot believed that sexual fluids had to be kept in careful balance and that masturbation put them out of balance and created ill health. He claimed that tuberculosis and other diseases that caused a weakening of the body were due to masturbation and that sexual activity damaged the nervous system, especially for women.

2. Sir Jonathan Hutchinson (1828–1913). In the late 1800s he published, *On Circumcision as Preventative of Masturbation,* which lead to many young men (and even some adult men) in England and the United States to be circumcised. Hutchinson basically started the modern practice of routine infant circumcision. His assertion that circumcision could stop masturbation caught on, and by 1920, a standard medical text in the United States said that having a foreskin would lead to wet dreams, hyperactivity, epilepsy, and "feeble-mindedness."

3. William Acton (1813–1875). Wrote *The Function and Disorders of the Reproductive Organs in Childhood, Youth, Adult Age and Advanced Life*, in 1857, which repeated the ideas of Tissot—that masturbation was responsible for the many ills of mankind. He wrote that when a boy masturbates he "shuns society of others, creeps about alone, joins with repugnance in the amusements of his school fellows. He cannot look anyone in the face, and becomes careless in dress and uncleanly in person. His intellect becomes sluggish and enfeebled."

4. Dr. Karl August Weinhold. In the Victorian era, English doctors created a way of stopping masturbation in young men called *infibulation*. During infibulation the boy's foreskin was pulled down, holes were punched in it, and it was laced tight. This prevented masturbation and made erections quite painful. In the 1820s, deep thinker Dr. Weinhold, a professor of surgery at the University of Halle, had a better idea. Why not use metal rings on the drawn-forward foreskin? These loops of wire could be covered with wax—if the wax became broken, the parent would know the boy had attempted masturbation. Weinhold performed this operation with great success, eventually suggesting that bachelors who were unlikely to marry be rounded up and fitted with such a wire, soldered permanently closed. In the 1870s he was able to carry out this plan in hospitals and mental institutions. "I mean," he said, "to go on wiring all masturbators."

5. Isaac Baker Brown (1812–1873). A British doctor who specialized in the removal of the clitoris, "either by scissors or knife—I always prefer the scissors." He believed that masturbation in women led to hysteria, epilepsy, and insanity—basically what all

11

these guys say. Clitorectomy was a preventative surgery that protected against these ills. He finally was stopped, not by moral outrage over what he was doing, but by the fact that he would promise to "cure" masturbation in women, but not tell them (or their husbands or families) what the cure entailed until the operation was over. He was ejected from the Obstetrical Society in 1867.

6. The Reverend Sylvester Graham. Graham was the inventor of the Graham cracker, originally a bland cracker that supposedly improved health and lowered sexual desires. Graham wrote the best-selling book, *A Lecture to Young Men* (1834), which told parents that a boy who masturbated would become a "degraded idiot, whose deeply sunken and vacant, glossy eye and livid shriveled countenance, and ulcerous, toothless gums, and fetid breath, and feeble broken voice, and emaciated and dwarfish and crooked body, and almost hairless head—covered perhaps with suppurating blisters and running sores—denote a premature old age!" With this fear in them, no wonder parents who listened to this popular sex expert went to hideous lengths to prevent their boys from masturbating.

Graham was a popular lecturer who told people how they could resist disease, including cholera, the epidemic of the day. His program had three principles—proper food (eat grains and avoid meat), exercises (males, especially, needed lots of strenuous exercise and were to sleep on hard wooden beds), and sexual abstinence (a never-ending quest). His contribution to this planet, aside from the Graham cracker, was that he did a lot to keep people hysterical and afraid about masturbation. He died in 1851, at the age of 57.

7. John Harvey Kellogg (1852–1943). At 24 years of age, in 1876, he became superintendent of the Adventist's Health Reform Institute, the Battle Creek (Michigan) Sanitarium. A Seventh-day Adventist and an ardent student of Graham's health techniques, Kellogg wrote his best-selling antimasturbation book, *Plain Facts for*

Old and Young Embracing the Natural History and Hygiene of Organic Life, on his honeymoon in 1888 (he was so committed to sexual abstinence he never consummated his relationship with his wife). Kellogg suggested and supported a variety of draconian methods of stopping masturbation: He suggested parents tie up their sons, put a cage over a child's genitals, or to have their boys circumcised without the aid of anesthetic. He also suggested that parents have boys' foreskins sutured shut, which would allow urination but prevent access to the glans, and make erections very painful. He thought that girls' parents should apply "pure carbolic acid to the clitoris." (See the list of antimasturbation devices for more on this.)

He discovered how to flake grains, thus inventing corn flakes in 1898—and they promptly became part of his diet plan for stopping sexual desire and masturbation. His younger brother, Will Keith Kellogg, added sugar to the flakes—thus making them useless, in John Harvey's opinion, for stopping masturbation. Will Keith Kellogg became a multimillionaire because of his brother's corn flake invention. John Harvey died poor in 1943 at the age of 91.

8. Anthony Comstock (1844–1915). Comstock served as a soldier in the Civil War, where he was shocked by *Fanny Hill* and the soldiers' morals. He became a crusader for public "decency," and was backed by wealthy J. Pierpont Morgan and Samuel Colgate. He successfully lobbied the U.S. Congress for passage of an act making it illegal to send pornography through the mails. President Grant appointed Comstock special agent of the Post Office Department, and his reign of terror began. He believed that information about contraception was obscene and suppressed it vigorously, as well as anything else he found objectionable. He remained special agent until his death in 1915, and the more draconian effects of the Comstock Act were not nullified until the 1950s.

*The only unnatural sex is that which
you cannot perform.*

—Alfred Kinsey

---◆---

"Obscene" Material Seized by the U.S. Postal Service Under the Comstock Act

The Comstock Act was passed by the U.S. Congress in 1873, and it gave Anthony Comstock far-reaching power to define and seize articles of obscenity. In the first six months of policing the U.S. Postal Service, Comstock seized:

1. 194,000 obscene pictures and photos

2. 134,000 pounds of obscene books

3. 14,200 stereopticon plates

4. 60,300 rubber items

5. 5,500 sets of obscene playing cards

6. 31,500 boxes of "aphrodisiacs"

*(I've convicted of obscenity) enough persons
to fill a passenger train of 61 coaches—
60 coaches containing 60 passengers and
the 61st not quite full.*

—Anthony Comstock

---◆---

14

J. H. Kellogg's Signs That a Young Man Might Be a Masturbator

J. H. Kellogg (the inventor of corn flakes) can help you tell if a young man is a masturbator. He'll have:

1. Rounded shoulders

2. Weak back

3. Stiffness of the joints

4. Paleness

5. Lack of breast development (in girls)

6. Acne

7. Heart palpitations

8. Fickleness

9. Bashfulness

10. Boldness

11. Confusion

12. Disgust at simple foods

13. Bed wetting

14. Nail biting

15. Consumption-like symptoms

16. Untrustworthiness

Masturbation! The amazing availability of it!

—James Joyce

———◆———

Antimasturbation Devices

From the late 1700s all the way into the 1930s, masturbation was considered an illness, leading to every disease and symptom of bad health on the planet. It wasn't just a few cranks who felt this way—

15

it was the prevailing opinion of doctors and all other health (and morality) experts, both in Europe and the United States. You could buy these antimasturbation devices in your local drugstore. Just as we say cigarette smoking is bad for you now (and make moral judgments about it), masturbation was the bugaboo of the past.

Between 1856 and 1932 the U.S. Government Patent Office awarded 33 patents to inventors of painful and humiliating devices to stop masturbation. Because no one was willing to admit that any sane adult man would masturbate, a disease was created to explain adult men's ejaculations—*spermatorrhea*—that was responsible for men's "involuntary" seminal emissions.

It's scary to contemplate the unquestionable fact that the people who created these devices considered themselves as intelligent and well meaning as we consider ourselves today. As one inventor of these torturous devices said, "I feel happy to have contributed my share to combating this pernicious evil."

1. Simple Bondage

Simply tying the masturbator up was often the solution parents used for masturbators. For example, in 1895 a girl of seven was thought to be masturbating, so she was made to sleep "in sheepskin pants and jacket made into one garment, with her hands tied to a collar about her neck; her feet were tied to the foot board and by a strap about her waist she was fastened to the headboard, so that she couldn't slide down in bed and use her heels; she had been reasoned with, scolded, and whipped, and in spite of it all she managed to keep up the habit."

2. Leather-Jacket Corset

A Dr. Fleck created a corset out of leather and steel for teenaged boys in 1831. In included a metal penis tube and "a steel band riveted to the shield permanently and attached to the

16

body with an encircling steel band in such a manner that it cannot be removed." It would "prevent access to the testicles with certainty."

"Thus equipped, the apparatus was applied to a 13-year-old boy in May 1831. After the boy had worn it a few weeks without adverse effect and without being able to produce an ejaculation, I was called because the patient complained of pain. I removed the machine, and found the penis enflamed and swollen, evidently because the penis tube was too small. After I had made a larger one, I placed the machine again on the patient. The boy wore the machine for another 16 days, when I was called again to his home. The patient had torn the steel bands from their attachment while in a secluded room and torn the silver shield as well, since the rivets failed to yield." After further modifications, the good doctor was able to report that "it closes with greatest accuracy, fits to perfection, and the boy wears it continuously without having succeeded even once in reaching his genitals or pulling the machine away from his body so as to produce friction on his genitals."

3. Spike-lined Ring

We now know that, in young boys, some nocturnal emissions are normal (as is masturbating). We also know that nocturnal erections are a natural part of the male sleep cycle. To prevent the nighttime display of sexuality, spike-lined penis rings were created by doctors in Boston in the early 1850s. In an 1854 edition of the respected medical journal *Lancet*, "spermatorrhea rings," as they were called, were glowingly discussed. The author, a doctor, explained that he had applied them "in hundreds of cases."

4. Spermatorrhea Bandage

Basically, spermatorrhea bandages were penis bondage. These bandages or devices kept the penis so tightly bound to the body that erection was impossible.

5. Stephenson Spermatic Truss

Some devices made sure the penis always pointed down, or strapped it between the legs to make erection impossible. One such device, the "Stephenson Spermatic Truss," was patented in 1876. The penis was placed in a pouch, then stretched and tied down and back between the legs, making erections extremely painful and masturbation impossible. He later created an improved version, out of wood. Another device, patented 21 years later, was a metal hood under which the penis could move freely, as long as it pointed downward. Any erection would drive the penis against painful spikes.

6. Bowen Device

This device, created in 1889 by James Bowen in Philadelphia, Pennsylvania, was like a cup or harness that fit over the head of the penis. It was attached to the pubic hair by chains and clips. If the wearer got an erection, the pubic hair would be pulled painfully. This would wake a sleeping patient, giving him the opportunity to "prevent or check the discharge."

7. The Cage

In 1885, the *Handbook of Medicine* mentions a metal cage that could be put around the genitals of a boy, allowing erections—which the inventor didn't deem as unhealthy—but preventing the boy from touching himself in any way. It was sold with handcuffs.

8. Dr. Moodie Apparatus for Boys

In 1848 Scotch physician John Moodie created a truss-and-shield to be attached to boys, with a penis tube that was closed at the end. There was a longitudinal slot on the side of the tube, which the boy had to push the end of his penis out of in order urinate—a position in which masturbation would be impossible. He also invented a panty girdle for girls, with an ivory grill over the genitals and a lock on the back, under a flap that would make any attempt to open it obvious.

9. Penis-Cooling Devices

These devices cooled the impending erection with either air or water. Because of their complexity, they were less popular than some of the other, more brute-force approaches. They were designed to prevent nocturnal erections and emissions. Frank Orth invented both water-cooled and air-cooled devices that were patented in 1893. They had electric motors, water reservoirs, and special undergarments a man would wear to bed, tethered to all this equipment. The creator said "the penis is inserted in the hole and between the levers," so that if "during the night an erection occurs, the dilation of the penis spreads the levers, thus separating the jaws, and permitting the cold water to flow through the tube to the sack or envelope. The cold water . . . cools the organ of generation, so that the erection subsides and no discharge occurs."

10. Sexual Armor

Invented by a Miss Perkins in 1908, the sexual armor was a jacket with leather pants, which support a large piece of steel armor. Perforations in the armor allowed urine to escape—if you wanted to defecate, you had to have someone else open the bolted, padlocked trapdoor at the rear. Miss Perkins was a nurse in a sanitarium. She created the armor because "it is a deplorable but well-known fact that one of the most common causes of insanity, imbecility and feeblemindedness, especially in youth, is due to masturbation or self-abuse. . . . Physicians, nurses and attendants associated with insane asylums have long found this habit the most difficult of all bad practices to eradicate, because of the incessant attention required of them in respect to the subjects in their care." Her "sexual armor" made this job easier.

No minister, moralist, teacher or scientific researcher has ever shown any evidence that masturbation is harmful in any way. Masturbation is fun.

—Dr. David Reuben

———◆———

11 Facts About Nazis and Sex

Few groups did a more complete job doing evil stuff than the Nazis. Their points of view on sex are less well-known than their other evil exploits.

1. In 1933 the Nazis adopted the Eugenic Sterilization Law. Under this law, *any* German citizen, not simply those in institutions, who had physical deformities, blindness, deafness, mental illness, or a host of other problems would be sterilized, so they could not breed further "imperfections" into the race. In response to charges that this was extremely cruel, one official said "We go beyond neighborly love, . . . We extend it to future generations. Therein lies the high ethical value and justification of the law."

2. In 1935 the Nazis passed a law outlawing not specific sex acts, but any sex act that respectable people might find improper.

3. The Marriage Law of 1935 prohibited persons with "hereditary illnesses" to marry. Once again, blindness, deafness, physical disability and mental illness were criteria, as well as behavioral problems created by "inferior genes." Emotional problems, nonconformity, poor work ethics, or delinquency also were suspect and could come under the sway of the law.

20

4. A 1935 decree called for the compulsory sterilization/castration of gay men, as well as other "degenerates," but many were not sterilized.

5. Nazi sex-education taught self-denial and discipline.

6. Men convicted of homosexual acts were sentenced to six-months' imprisonment, often followed by being sent to concentration camps. They were forced to wear pink triangles.

7. It is estimated that 50,000 homosexual men were sent to concentration camps; tens of thousands of them died there.

8. Nazi laws against homosexuality did not proscribe lesbianism, though lesbian behavior could be prosecuted under other laws.

9. Elite Nazi women went to the Women's Academy of Wisdom and Culture. Only blue-eyed, attractive women were allowed. They were trained to be the future mothers of the pure German race, wives to the Nazi elite.

10. Elite SS troops were not allowed to have sex with any women other than German women—any man breaking this rule was reported directly to Heinrich Himmler.

11. Hitler sought to combat prostitution by encouraging early marriage.

*Homosexuality is assuredly no advantage,
but it is nothing to be ashamed of,
no vice, no degradation, it cannot be
classified as an illness.*

—Sigmund Freud

Sex Gods and Goddesses
in Various Cultures

Most religious traditions have gods and goddesses who are venerated around sex, love, eroticism, birth, and fertility, both for people and for the harvest. Here are some historic gods and goddesses that had to do with sex, so you know whom to call upon next time you need a little sexual help:

1. **Aztec and Mayan**
   Tlazolteotl. Goddess of Lust (Aztec)
   Itzamna. God of Fertility (Mayan)

2. **Assyro-Babylonian**
   Ishtar. Goddess of Love and War
   Ninurta. God of Fertility and of War
   Tammuz. God of the Harvest

3. **Chinese**
   Chi-nu. Spinster Goddess
   Hsi-wang-mu. Mother Goddess
   Kuan-Yin. Goddess of Health and Fertility

4. **Egyptian**
   Hathor. Goddess of Love
   Isis. Goddess of Beauty
   Min. Phallic God

5. **Greek**
   Apollo. God of Beauty and Light
   Aphrodite. Goddess of Love and Beauty
   Artemis. Goddess of the Moon, Childbirth
   Gaea. Earth Goddess
   Hera. Goddess of Motherhood and Marriage
   Priapos. God of the Phallus

6. **Indian**
   Kali. Mother Goddess, Goddess of Destruction
   Lakshmi. Goddess of Love and Beauty
   Shiva. Phallic God of Fertility, Creation, and Destruction

7. **Japanese**
   Benzaiten. Goddess of Love
   Chimata-no-Kami. Phallic God
   Kishi-mojin. Goddess of Childbirth

8. Phoenician
Adonis. God of Fertility
Baalat. Mother Goddess
Mot. God of the Harvest

9. Roman
Apollo. God of Beauty and Light
Bacchus. God of Wine and Inspiration
Cupid. God of Love
Diana. Goddess of Hunting, the Moon, Childbirth
Juno. Goddess of Marriage
Mars. God of War and Fertility
Mercury. God of Fertility
Priapus. God of the Phallus
Venus. Goddess of Beauty and Love

Cupid is a knavish cad,
Thus to make poor females mad.

—William Shakespeare

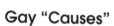

Gay "Causes"

It's taken a long time for people to figure out that life is actually easier if one lives with most sexual preferences, rather than trying to cure them. Homosexuality, especially, has been scrutinized extensively for "causes" and "cures." Here's a list of the most popular reasons men were thought to become gay:

• Demonic possession

• Planetary and astrological influences

• A domineering mother

• An overly passive, distant father

• Hormonal imbalance—too much estrogen, too little testosterone

- Genetics

- Being warned/trained against being sexual with the opposite sex

- Having a gay pastor or teacher

- Liking, disliking, identifying with, or not identifying with either parent

- Shame about a mother's or sister's promiscuity

- Homosexuality taken on to degrade or humiliate resented parents

- Parent's heterosexual relationship was unhappy, set a bad example

- Sister was liked by parents more than he, so he tries to be like his sister

- Convenience of casual homosexual sex

- Easier to get love from members of the same sex

- Have more in common with members of the same sex

- Early trauma with a girlfriend

- Shame about being male, or about what men have done

- Shortage of suitable women, as in frontier settings, prison, or at the South Pole (ratio: 1 woman to 250 men—"there are no unattractive women at the South Pole")

- Masturbation (Of course, if this made everybody who did it gay, wouldn't we all be?)

- A "too small" hypothalamus (from a controversial 1991 study by Simon LeVay)

- Prenatal influences (Mom smoke, drank, did drugs, which affected the developing fetus.)

- Having gay role models as a child

- Having early pleasurable sexual experiences with other boys
- Not having prostitutes to have sex with, so therefore turning to other males. No lesser personages than St. Augustine and St. Aquinas made this strange argument.

Ten percent of all men are, more or less, exclusively homosexual for at least three years between the ages of 16 and 55.

—Alfred Kinsey

Lesbian "Causes"

Here's a list of the most popular reasons women were thought to become lesbians:

- Masturbation (blamed for pretty much everything, pretty much throughout history)
- Failing nervous system (1800s)
- Shortage of men (after major wars)
- Genetic brain problems (1800s)
- Feminism (late 1800s, 1960s)
- Women's athletics (early 1900s)
- Glandular problems, especially adrenal problems (1930s–1950s)
- Associating overmuch with males (1800s)
- Associating overmuch with females (1800s)
- Traumatic experiences in youth (1920s—present)
- Parent's fault (1960s)

*All women are lesbians, except those
who don't know it yet.*

—Jill Johnson

Gay "Cures" in History

1. Testicular castration

2. Electroshock therapy

3. X-raying glands (to correct hypothesized "glandular imbalance")

4. Lobotomy—seems to be everybody's favorite, a way to limit sexual desires, as well as limiting memory, speech, and emotion

5. Libido inhibitors—that is, the use of female sex hormones in men, especially estrogens, such as stilbestrol. Done too long, though, it produces chemical castration. Whoops!

6. Narcoanalysis—using a sedative plus psychotherapy

7. Hypnosis

8. Sedation

9. Behavioral therapy—associate pain with homosexual thoughts, pleasure with heterosexual

10. Systematic desensitization

11. Changing the environment—taking the person out of the "gay world"

Most of my male friends are gay, and that seems perfectly natural to me. I mean, who wouldn't like cock?

—Valerie Perrine

Lesbian "Cures" in History

Some of the "cures" for lesbianism are laughable, others are downright draconian.

1. Rest, visiting a spa (late 1800s)

2. Making girls wear dresses and behave like girls (early 1900s)

3. Segregating girls from boys (early 1900s)

4. Being sure *not* to segregate girls from boys (also early 1900s)

5. Not allowing girls to sleep in the same bed (early 1900s)

6. Finding religion, being "cured," followed by being on the cover of *Newsweek* (1990s)

7. Willpower (always)

8. Therapy (1930s–1970s)

9. Increased stress on religion (always)

10. Lesbian "deprogramming" (1950s–1980s)

11. Hospitalization in mental hospitals (1930s–1970s)

12. Bromides (1860s)

13. Anaphrodisiacs (these are the *opposite* of aphrodisiacs— *anaphrodisiacs* decrease all sexual desire) (late 1800s)

14. Male hormones (1950s)

15. Hormone injections (1930s)

16. Surgical removal of the ovaries (oöpherectomy) (late 1800s)

17. Surgical removal of the clitoris (clitoridectomy) (mid 1800s)

What did Lesbian Sappho teach girls but love?

—Ovid

Devilish Sex: Historic Rumors, Facts, and Tidbits About Sex with the Devil

There have been claims and reports of women, and occasionally men, having sex with the devil and demonic images for centuries. Historically, there have been primarily two types of devil. The *incubus* and the *succubus*. The incubus refers to a male devil and the succubus is the female devil. Both are popular in reports of devil sex. It is thought that the church created myths about sex with the devil in an attempt to bring charges against innocent men and women during the Inquisition. Here are a few other facts and rumors on this matter:

1. Witches claimed that they had sex with devils during sabbats.

2. Theologians who believed in the devil, believed that he would visit and prey upon women while they were sleeping.

3. Thomas Aquinas had a theory about the inner workings of the succubus. He claimed that the devil wanted to have a child and would change himself into a succubus in order to copulate. He would then turn into an incubus and implant his sperm into the succubus. Yes, it makes no sense to us either.

4. During the Inquisition, starting in 1430, many women were persecuted for having sexual relations with devils. Sometimes girls as young as nine were persecuted.

5. It is noted that in 1628 in Wurzburg, Germany, several girls aged eight to twelve claimed to have had sex with an incubus. The oldest girl was sentenced to death.

6. It is estimated that over 300 children claimed to have had sex with devils.

7. Several satanic cults conduct a ritual whereby a high-ranking man dresses as a devil wearing a horned mask as well as black robes and unusual leather shoes. He then recites some prayers and has sexual intercourse with several women while other cult members watch. This ritual is said to be modeled after stories of the incubus.

8. Faust wrote several stories about a succubus.

9. Many women who have had sexual experiences with incubi claim that the penises of such devils are cold and are shaped like icicles. Other women claim sperm from incubi are freezing cold.

10. Some ancient authorities claimed that the devil frequently appeared as an animal, often as a goat, bird or raven. The devil would then try to seduce innocent men into having sex with them because bestiality was even more taboo.

11. In 1679 several Scottish witches claimed that the devil would seduce them while taking the form of a dog or deer.

12. It is said that in 1566 several nuns had sex with a devil while the devil was in the form of a dog.

13. Some demonologists believed that the incubi would steal semen from corpses.

14. Pope Sylvester II (999–1003) was said to engage in sorcery. It is reported that he had several sexual encounters with a succubus named Meridiana. She was known to frequently appear in his bed in spirit form.

15. Other demonologists believed that incubi would visit men while they were sleeping and force them into having nocturnal emissions.

16. Criminals have often told judges that the devil forced them to rape women and to commit crimes. In the 1400s this type of defense was acceptable and often successful.

The good news is that Jesus is coming back. The bad news is that He's really pissed off.

—Bob Hope

---◆---

History of Birth Control

1700s: The Dutch-Cap was used for birth control. A half of a lemon was used as a cervical cap for women.

Late 1700s: Casanova popularizes an early version of the condom.

1806: Dr. Ewell suggests that couples "copulate in vessels filled with carbonic acid or azotic gas" as a birth-control method.

1838: Infanticide is proposed for family planning.

1847: Goodyear discovers a way to vulcanize rubber, leading to the production of rubber condoms.

1882: Aletta Jacobs opens first birth control clinic.

1883: Diaphragm is invented.

1883: First vasectomy is performed.

1909: First IUD invented in Germany.

1910: Margaret Sanger begins promoting birth control in New York.

1930: Research is published that shows the success rate of the IUD.

1930: Researchers show the validity of the rhythm method.

1951: First version of the pill is created by Carl Djerassi.

1960: FDA approves the pill.

1963: IUD becomes widely available.

1973: The landmark case, *Roe vs. Wade,* essentially made abortion legal and protected abortion rights.

1970s: Depo-provera injections become available in 50 nations (though not in the United States until 1992).

1988: The cervical cap is approved by the FDA.

1990: Norplant is first available.

1992: The pill RU-486 is made available in France, China, and England. This pill can be taken up to nine weeks after conception and will successfully remove an embryo. This pill is still not available in the United States.

1994: Female condom is introduced.

*There's the Greek method. Apparently one can
temporarily sterilize oneself by heating one's
organs in boiling water.*

—Annon. British Teenager,
from Michael Schofield,
Sexual Behavior of Young People

---◆---

The History of the Dildo

The sex toy and masturbation device known as the dildo has a rich
history. It has been used for hundreds of years to inspire the masturbation fantasies of millions of people. Dildos were often manufactured in secrecy, as they were often illegal. Dildos have been
made from a variety of media, from stone and wood, to the current
use of latex to clay and everything in between. Today mechanical
stimulators are very popular. It is estimated that nearly 10 percent
of American women have used one at some point in their lives.
Wanna know more? Read on:

1. In 500 B.C. leather and wood sex toys became popular. The
   demand was so great that they had to set up factories in
   Turkey to satisfy the demand.

2. Arab and Polynesian women used bananas as dildos.

3. Throughout the Middle Ages hand-crafted penises were
   marketed and distributed throughout Europe.

4. In Ancient Rome a wooden penis created in the name of fertility god Liber was used to deflower women soon to be married.

5. In the eighteenth century Europe's upper-class women
   demanded dildos for their personal use. Several new forms

of dildos emerged at this time. They were made from silver and ivory and contained internal chambers that could be filled with warm water for extra stimulation.

6. In nineteenth-century Uganda, brides had to be deflowered before they could have sex with a king. His court created several artificial phalluses made from metal, stone, and ivory.

7. Havelock Ellis noticed that wealthy women in India, China, and Japan had used stimulators for vaginal masturbation for many years.

8. There were several sexual foods eaten by would-be brides and barren wives. They ate *Mandelchen*, an oblong cookie made of almond paste and topped with two nuts to represent testicles. They also ate *Liebesknochen*, which translates as "the bone of love." It was a thick, vanilla-cream-filled dessert that looked like a phallus. Another type of dessert they ate was called a *Vielliebchen*, or "much love." This was also a long phallus-shaped dessert with cream in the middle. It also had two nuts on the top to represent testicles.

9. In 1899 American doctors popularized new vibrators that were pressurized by hose units.

10. In 1907 the *Liquid Actuated Vibrator* was patented. It had a nubbed head for clitoral stimulation.

11. In 1911 the first electrical dildo was sold.

12. In 1966 the one-piece, battery-powered, vibrating dildo was patented. This was to become the best-selling dildo of all time.

13. Another dildo breakthrough happened in 1968 when the battery pack was held in place by a waist strap.

14. In the 1960s the first male stimulators hit the market.

15. In 1964 a vibrating collar designed to wrap around the penis was sold.

16. In 1975 a huge tabletop sized machine called the "hydraulic orgasm machine" was patented. It featured a large vagina sleeve.

You know it's lust when you satisfy your real needs. It's when you need nothing else, except the feeling of it.

—Sandra Bernhard

Breast Implants: A Brief History

The first breast implants were designed in the 1950s by scientists. They were made of silicone and designed for women to insert into their bras to enhance their breast size. The first real implant was done by plastic surgeons Thomas Cronin and Frank Gerow in 1962. Over the next decade companies such as Dow Corning and other scientific manufacturing companies created their own implants. By 1973 over 50,000 women had implants. However, there were several problems; implants leaked, and some women were developing medical problems. Dow Corning attempted to correct the problems by developing a water based version.

Here are some other moments in breast implant history of interest to all:

1947: After WWII Japanese prostitutes who were servicing American GIs searched for ways to increase their breast size because they thought they could then charge more money.

The first implants were made from saline solution. Then doctors experimented with goat's milk. Then they tried paraffin wax. None of these worked well.

1977: The first successful implant suit was a jury case. The woman whose implants ruptured was awarded $170,000 in damages.

1982: The first report of connective tissue pain attributed to implants is noted in Australia.

1984: The first case alleging autoimmune disease due to implants is won.

1988: The FDA becomes involved and requires manufacturers to prove the safety of implants.

1991: The largest judgment to date for an implant case is awarded. A woman is awarded $7.34 million in a jury case.

1992: A Texas jury awards a woman $25 million, the largest judgment to date.

1994: Dow Corning and other companies offer a $4.25 billion settlement to women who have had breast-implant surgery.

1995: Dow Corning files for bankruptcy.

2000: Adjustable implants, whose size can be easily changed by an office visit to the doctor, hit the market.

Everybody knows I've got bigger boobs than Carol Burnett.

—Julie Andrews

———◆———

Phallic Statues and Symbols

In our culture the idea of a phallic statue is humorous. We are not ones to idealize or canonize the idea of phallic stature. In many cultures around the world the penis was worshipped as was the vagina. There were sperm cults and fertility rites, phallic worship, and goddess worship. In Asia many households had small phallic statues on their altars. Penis statues were popular up until the 1800s. Penis parades still take place in Japan each year. These traditions are at least interesting and at best inspiring.

1. In Japan, *Dosojin* sculptures are part of the folk religious tradition. It is noted that Dosojin carved sculptures that were phallic in nature. Researchers found over 3,000 of these stones. Many are approximately two feet tall and hundreds are over five feet tall.

2. Small phallic statues have been found by archeologists in Argentina and Brittany.

3. Cave drawings were the first to display phallic art. Many of the men depicted had large and erect penises. A large penis was said to be linked to cosmic power.

4. Many people claim that European clock towers not only look like phallic statues, but they are in fact phallic statues. Around Europe it is traditional for these towers to be found in the middle of cemeteries. Many older civilizations worshiped the phallus and would build tall representations as a sign of respect.

5. During the fifteenth century the Kacharis tribe erected more than 30 phallic statues on the India-Burma border. Each statue was over 20 feet high.

6. The Empire State Building is considered by some to be a phallic statue.

7. In 1955 a team of archeologists in Corsica discovered several phallic monuments dating back to the Bronze Age. Each statue was at least ten feet tall.

8. There were many phallic statues carved during the Stone Age period.

9. Many ancient tribes wore phallic jewelry.

10. Researchers claim that in parts of Africa phallic statues were made of black stone, and oil was placed on them to appease the Phallic gods.

11. In Yucatan there are many phallic statues. In some areas there are rows of statues nearly eight feet tall.

12. The Ancient Greeks had a huge penis celebration called *phallophoriai.*

13. Phallic statues were often made with rough stone; smoothed stones were saved for vaginal statues.

14. In Ireland phallic statues have been linked to Pagan and Druid religions.

15. Several phallic statues are known to have been erected during the Neolithic Period, approximately 2000 B.C.

16. Sixty-five phallic statutes have been identified in Ireland, mostly in Kildare. The tallest statue is 90 feet high with a circumference of 48 feet.

17. There is a class of phallic stone statues called *menhir.* They have ritual symbolism and are usually created to invoke power and protection.

A man is two people, himself and his cock.
A man always takes his friend to the party.
Of the two, the friend is the nicer, being
able to show his feelings.

—Beryl Bainbridge

———◆———

Chastity Belts: 18 Historical Facts and Myths

Chastity belts were used on women to ensure that they were not cheating on their husbands. They were also used as anti-masturbation devices. Chastity belts became popular in the fifteenth and sixteenth centuries across Europe. These devices were often quite painful to wear and showed a common disrespect for women. Many chastity belts contained padlocks and were used by husbands as a form of domination, torture, and humiliation. Some recent authors note that these belts look more like safety-deposit boxes on a leather strap than a torture device. The history of chastity belts also contains moments when these belts were fashionable and worn for decoration rather than for control.

1. Chastity belts were first used in the fourteenth century in Italy. References have been made to similar devices since as early as 1150, during the Crusades.

2. In Paris, France, some women were forced to wear iron chastity belts. One in particular consisted of an iron hoop that was covered with velvet. The iron hoop had notches so that the man could tighten and loosen it depending on his mood. In the front of the belt was an ivory panel that cov-

ered the pubic area. There was a very narrow area left open for urination and menstruation.

3. In 1406 Novella Carrara was put to death. Carrara was a much despised Venetian known for being cruel and oppressive. He had forced his wife to wear a metal chastity belt that included sharp teeth around the inside of the device near her anus and vulva.

4. Chastity belts were often made in only one size. Larger women were forced to wear them and suffer the pain from the tight fit.

5. In the sixteenth and seventeenth centuries a popular belt in Central Europe was the iron girdle, which had a circumference of 80 centimeters. The area surrounding the hips was made of four metal bands. There were small holes for urination, and the entire device was kept in place by a padlock.

6. In Rome female slaves were forced to wear chastity belts that would readily expose their genitalia for the sexual pleasure of their masters.

7. In 1930 several women were reportedly seen wearing chastity belts in the Middle East by the U.S. military.

8. In 1848 a respected doctor in Scotland wrote a book in which he supported the use of chastity belts on both men and women as a means to prevent masturbation and preserve chastity and morality. In his book he shows how to manufacture chastity belts step-by-step.

9. During the fourth century Roman maidens were forced to wear woolen girdles. Wool was used to excite love. The girdle was also tied with a special "Herculean knot."

10. The Marquis de Sade was a known lover of chastity belts. He forced all his lovers to wear them.

11. Roman and Greek women often wore metal or leather belts over their gowns or dresses. Other styles included single, crisscross, double, and triple belts. These styles were all worn to draw attention to the woman's breasts and hips.

12. Roman prostitutes were sometimes forced to wear chastity belts. They wore the belts to brothels. There was one hitch, however—the belts revealed their pubic region and were worn to tempt male customers into being more interested in hiring them for sex. The men running the brothels would then be contacted to take off the belts and collect the money. They could then know exactly how much money was being taken in by each prostitute.

13. In one Sudanese harem a particularly brutal chastity belt was used. This included a bamboo stick, which was inserted into the vagina. It was held in place by a strap with another shield covering the vulva. The entire thing went around the hips and waist and was secured by a padlock. A eunuch controlled the key and was left to guard over the many members of the harem.

14. In 1897 an American inventor patented a chastity belt that had a metal shield covering the abdomen and was held together by a lock in the back. The device also had a hole large enough for a penis to be inserted.

15. One of the most unusual chastity belts is on display at the Cluny Museum in Paris. It includes over a dozen hinges and crude iron drawers covering each part of the woman's pelvis. As usual a narrow opening was included for urination.

16. Throughout the nineteenth century many women were forced to wear "day belts" when they went on unsupervised trips or when traveling.

17. To this day no law exists to prohibit the manufacture or use of chastity belts.

18. In recent decades chastity belts have been used by men and women involved in bondage fantasies. Modern belts are made of leather and steel.

A woman who has once lost chastity has lost every good quality. She has from that moment all the vices.

—Josephine Butler, 1896, from her book,
Personal Reminances of a Great Crusade

---◆---

24 Writers, Researchers, Artists, and Performers Who Reformed Sex

Many of the people on this list experienced much hardship, sometimes jail terms, because they spoke out about sexuality. They pushed barriers and broke laws to move sexuality to the next level of social understanding and acceptability. Much of the sexual freedom and understanding, not to mention the widespread availability of sex, we experience is because of the groundbreaking work of many of these people.

1. William Burroughs

He was one of the first openly homosexual authors. Burroughs' books portrayed the life of a junkie, sex freak, and beat writer. His book *The Wild Boys* published in 1971 was one of the first to describe homosexual sex in great detail. He died in 1999.

2. Betty Dodson

Dodson was one of the first women to write and discuss female masturbation. Dodson even put on masturbation seminars for women. Her book *Liberating Masturbation* brought a new level of self-awareness to women. She has also been an active sex educator and activist since the 1970s.

3. Havelock Ellis

Ellis was one of the first sex researchers. He began his work even before Kinsey. His seminal book *The Psychology of Sex* was a groundbreaking source of sex information. Ellis died in 1939 in England.

4. Federico Fellini

His films were some of the first to include overtly erotic images. Films such as *La Dolce Vita* and *Juliet of the Spirits* inspired a new wave of sexuality and art.

5. Sigmund Freud

Whether you hate the guy or not he was one of the original sex therapists and researchers examining the role of sexuality in the functioning of the psyche. He opened many doors—and made many mistakes in the process.

6. Bob Guccione

Guccione was the first person to take pornography to a new level of respectability. While Hugh Heffner was brave enough to bring *Playboy* to the public, Guccione founded *Penthouse*, which brought hardcore pornography to mainstream America.

7. Radclyffe Hall

This Italian novelist wrote and published the first lesbian novel entitled *The Well of Loneliness* in 1928.

8. Xaviera Hollander

This Dutch woman was one of the most outspoken erotica writers of the twentieth century. She authored a series of popular books and remains a legend.

9. Erica Jong

She is the author of the book *Fear of Flying*, which was published in 1977. Jong was one of the first to bring explicit sexuality into popular fiction. She also created the phrase "zipless fuck."

10. W. H. Auden

He wrote many erotic poems and stories. He wrote several poems about homosexuality that became popular in the 1970s.

11. Robert Crumb

This cartoonist was one of the first to create explicit cartoon strips. He is well known for his depiction of women with large breasts and large bodies. Before Crumb there were very few sexual cartoons. He has been a major influence on sexual art since 1974.

12. Alfred Kinsey

Kinsey was the first person to conduct large-scale sex-research surveys. During his career he interviewed over 17,000 people. His groundbreaking work on sexuality altered popular views about what can be considered normal and abnormal sexual behavior. The Kinsey Institute, the largest establishment of its kind, is still in existence and houses one of the largest collections of sexual books in the world. Kinsey died in 1956.

13. The Mitchell Brothers

These brothers were sex pioneers in the 1970s. They opened the largest and most extravagant sex theatre, the O'Farrel, in San Francisco. They also produced several groundbreaking sex films starring Marilyn Chambers. They were some of the first to create strip clubs that were plush and accessible.

14. Robert Mapplethorpe

This cult photographer was one of the first to include gay and S/M photos in his collection. He was one of the most beloved photographers of our time. Mapplethorpe was banned by the NEA after a photo exhibit in Ohio that contained a photo of a man urinating on another man. He was a gifted photographer that revolutionized sexual and erotic photography. He died of AIDS after his first exhibit in New York at the Whitney Museum.

15. William Masters and Virginia Johnson

These sex researchers were some of the first to conduct scientific experiments that measured sexual stimulation, particularly female orgasm. Their research helped create the field of sex therapy and sexual surrogates.

16. Sheikh Nefzawi

This Islamic author wrote *The Perfumed Garden* in the fifteenth century. His book has become a classic sex text throughout the world. Many claim that his work is as important as the *Kama Sutra* for studying sexual techniques.

17. Anaïs Nin

She was born in 1903 in France and has become one of the most celebrated authors of erotica in history. Nin was one of the first women to publish erotica and is popular still. She had a long affair with author Henry Miller and is known to be his major influence in his writing career. Her numerous books include *Little Birds* and *Delta of Venus*.

18. Betty Page

Page is one of the unsung heroes of the world of sex symbols. Page was a popular fetish model in the 1950s and 1960s. She was one of the first to appear nude and in lingerie. The United States government later banned her pictures and films. She went bankrupt and disappeared from the spotlight.

19. Wilhelm Reich

Reich was an Austrian psychologist who was a groundbreaking sex researcher. He researched sexual energy and opened up the field of bioenergetics. Later in his career he created the *Orgone Box*, a device used to measure and expand sexual energy. He also helped to set up sex-hygiene clinics in Vienna. He then moved to Berlin where psychologists banned his work. Reich was one of the first to lobby for sexual rights. During his life he faced much opposition, yet continued to publish his work and fight for what he believed was right.

20. Leopold von Sacher Masoch

This seventeenth-century author is famous for writing the book *Venus in Furs*. He was the first author to write about S/M. Much of the history of kinky sex comes from his notes and his published work.

21. Henri de Toulouse-Lautrec

Lautrec was a nineteenth-century painter who created many erotic prints. He was known for painting prostitutes. He lived in a brothel for a period. Lautrec was able to bring beauty and dignity to an art form previously considered lewd.

22. Pandit Vatsyayana

He is credited with writing the *Kama Sutra* between the first and the fourth centuries. He researched many ancient Indian texts and was able to create the most widely popular system for sexuality and sexual positions ever to be published.

23. Leonardo da Vinci

This Italian artist popularized the human form through his work. He produced many paintings featuring genitalia and sexual intercourse. His work was banned at various periods in history.

24. Oscar Wilde

This popular Irish playwright was a homosexual socialite and activist. He went on trial for homosexual behavior in 1896 and was in jail for a year. Wilde popularized gay humor and was able to interject homosexuality into his many plays. Wilde's work continues to be popular in theaters around the world.

La Dolce Vita (1959) was Federico Fellini's exposé of "the sweet life," a sprawling persuasive orgiastic movie assumed by many to have contributed to a decline in standards because it reported without condemning.

—Leslie Halliwell

---◆---

Great Moments in Corset History

Few other items have more erotic connotation than the corset. It has been used both as a sexual torture device as well as an erotic teaser from women for many centuries. Corsets have been used to temporarily or permanently reshape a woman's torso. Many women claim that wearing a corset is in itself an erotic experience. To examine the corset is to not only look at the history of women's undergarments, but also to explore sexual fashions.

1. Some experts claim that the first corsets were worn in Africa by the Dinka to rearrange the body and make it more attractive.

2. In the Dinka tradition each corset is beaded. The color of the beads is an indicator of age. For example, red and black

beads are worn by the 15 to 25 year olds, pink
and purple by those 25 to 30, and everyone over 30 wears
yellow.

3. Young men who lived in islands near Crete wore belts similar to corsets. They wore them to see how small they could
compress their waists.

4. Early tribes wore corsets because it was useful in teaching
them to ignore their bodies, so they could be more fierce in
combat. It was also a spiritual experience designed so that
the boys wearing the belts would have to transcend their
temporal experience.

5. The first corset is seen in a collection of drawings done in
the twelfth century by Sir John Cotton. In the drawings a
devil is shown with a woman's body. She has a bird type body,
but is wearing an unusual skirt that is long and has several
knots from the bottom to the top.

6. In the seventeenth century it is rumored that Napoleon and
the British Army employed waist training as a military method.

7. Medieval fashions for women were anything but revealing.
However, by 1790 the corset appeared.

8. The word "corset" appeared in the English language in 1887.

9. Early corsets were made of rose-pink watered silk.

10. In 1795 a newspaper article denounced corsets as being too
revealing.

11. Many famous artists and writers of the early 1800s were
against the corset. Leonardo da Vinci wrote that he was
concerned that women would suffocate from wearing
them.

12. After the initial public shock about corsets, manufacturers began making shorter corsets that prominently emphasized the waist and breasts.

13. By 1810 many mothers were encouraging their daughters to wear these fashionable items. Mothers often had to help their daughters put on the corset by holding the girl on the floor and putting her foot into the daughters back to tighten the laces.

14. While corsets were considered sexy in their day, they were quite large in comparison with today's version. They generally came high above the waist and covered the breasts.

15. In the 1830s the rubber industry changed corsets with the advent of new closure devices. They also helped corset makers to invent "bust improvers," which were rubber devices that could be inserted into the corset to increase the appearance of the wearer's breasts.

16. It is difficult to become pregnant when a woman has a tiny waist. Some women found that the corset helped them to achieve liberation.

17. By the 1860s there was wide public controversy about the safety of corsets. Queen Victoria was opposed to them.

18. In 1870 corsets started to be worn extra tightly. Many public figures thought that tightly worn garments were good. There was even a book written in favor of this entitled *The Corset and the Crinoline*, by William Barry Lord.

19. In 1870 several English citizens claimed that the corset was a form of pornography. Samual Beeton lead the fight against the corset claiming that it was a form of perversion.

20. In Germany experts discouraged women from wearing corsets because they claimed that they could lead to liver damage.

21. By 1880 a softer-looking corset was being made from silks, satin, and lace.

22. In 1890 a Frenchman made corset history when he patented a woven corset on a loom. These were the first corsets made for widespread distribution.

23. The next important change in corsets came in the 1930s with the invention of elastic. The new look and feel was more comfortable and relaxed.

24. In 1917 French actress Mademoiselle Polaire was seen with a 14-inch waist. She was an avid corset advocate.

25. In 1944 the Corset Guild of Great Britain was formed. They eventually established the "Essential Works Order," which created industry standards on the production of corsets.

26. In 1945 Dr. Jaeuger created the "health corset," which was designed to increase female health and fitness. This corset was designed to leave the thorax free while supporting the abdomen.

27. The most famous corseted woman of all time is Ethel Granger. She had a 13-inch waist. Her nose and nipples were pierced. She worked at a corset shop in London and died at age 83.

28. In several movies from the 1950s, such as *Cat on a Hot Tin Roof* and *Raintree County*, Elizabeth Taylor is seen wearing corsets.

When undressing, when arising, be mindful of modesty and take care not to expose to others anything that morality and nature require to be concealed.

—Desiderius Erasmus, *Adagia*
(Sixteenth Century)

———◆———

The Chronological History of Love

The word "love" was first used in the English language around 1157. We have traced many common and uncommon phrases containing the word love and when it was first introduced into the English vocabulary.

1. **Lovely:** First introduced in 1200; meaning beautiful or attractive

2. **Lovesome:** 1245; meaning affectionate, desirable or sexy

3. **Love-knot:** 1327; a specific knot made from a chain or other type of jewelry that was an emblem of love

4. **Lovesick:** 1400s; longing for love and yearning

5. **Love-making:** 1400s; dealing with courtship and copulation

6. **Love-feast:** 1580; a gathering to honor a loved one or to reconcile after a fight

7. **Love-affair:** 1591; referring to a romantic episode

8. **Lovelies:** 1652; referring to two or more beautiful women

9. **Love score:** 1800s; a tennis expression meaning zero

10. **Love child:** 1805; an illegitimate child

11. **Loving cup:** 1812; an ornamental mug with two or more handles and used for ceremonial toasting

12. **Lovey-dovey:** 1886; a loving and sentimental expression, also known as a mushy phrase

13. **Love seat:** 1902; at the turn of the century this was the most common type of sofa. It was designed for two people to sit comfortably at one time

14. **Love-bug:** 1966; the nickname for the Volkswagen Beetle

15. **Love-in:** 1967; a gathering of people for sex or for love

16. **Love-beads:** 1968; referring to strings of beads used to symbolize love and peace

17. **Love handles:** 1975; used as a nickname for the fatty bulges on a man's stomach a woman can grab during sex

Love is a universal migraine,
A bright stain on the vision
Blotting out reason.

—Robert Graves, *Symptoms of Love*

———◆———

Bra History

Ancient China: A very early precursor to the bra was used by women to cover their breasts so that their husbands would not see bite marks made by an illegitimate lover.

1840s: Corsets were popularized; Olivia P. Flynt, a Boston dressmaker patented a precursor to the bra called the "bust supporter."

1897: A rubber bra was manufactured by George McCleary.

1898: A Deadwood, South Dakota man invented the "breast shield," designed to support, augment, and keep the breasts warm in the winter.

The "bust bodice" came into fashion in France.

1912: The word "brassiere" was noted by the Oxford dictionary.

Mary Phelps Jacobs patented the first bra.

1914: The "backless bra" was invented.

1920s: The brassiere was popularized. It was seen by women as a symbol of physical and social freedom.

1921: Mary Phelps Jacobs sold her bra patent to the Warner Brothers Corset Company for $1,500.

1920s–30s: Mae West popularized the pointed bust and exaggeration of bust shape in film.

1932: Bra-slips were first produced.

1935: The word "bra" became a popular expression for the brassiere.

Warner Brothers introduced cup fittings for bras (A, B, C, and D were used).

1944: A wraparound bra made of soft material was made to accommodate several sizes and shapes of breasts.

1947: Etta Harvey of Pennsylvania invented a bra with zippered pockets designed to hold money.

A United States man invented a bra that had holes around the nipples so that they could be prominently noticed.

Mid 1900's: The breasts were a major focus in women's apparel

1949: Iver Hill invented the strapless bra.

The wired bra hit the marketplace.

1950: An inventor from Georgia created a bra with rubber cups designed to enhance the appearance and size of the breasts.

1950s: The inflatable bra hit the market.

1957: The "sweater bra" was popularized by Jane Russell.

1959: A bra with electric nipple stimulators was patented.

1964: Training bras hit the marketplace.

1970s: Bras were designed for comfort. They began to be manufactured with knitted weaves, sheer and clinging fabrics, and were naturally shaped.

1974: The first international symposium on garment-apparel industry technologists took place in Atlanta, Georgia, and was attended by more than 270 people.

1976: The T-shirt bra was popularized.

1977: The first molded panty/corset appeared.

1977: Molded bras were becoming popular, and lycra, polyester, and knitted simplex were used.

There is not upon earth so impertinent a thing as women's modesty.

—Sir John Vanbrugh (1664–1726)

———◆———

Superstitions and Myths About
Menstruation and Menstrual Blood

1. Some cultures believed that the blood lost by a woman possesses magic properties, both evil and dangerous.

2. Several religions, to this day, forbid men from having sex with a menstruating woman.

3. Ancient Greek culture believed that when a woman is having her menstrual period she is under the influence of demons.

4. Several cultures believed that menstrual blood is a medical cure for gout, dog bites, smallpox, and leprosy.

5. In the 1700s it was a popular belief in Europe that menstrual blood from a virgin could cure any disease.

6. Several books on witchcraft mention that dried menstrual blood worn in an amulet could prevent the plague and other diseases.

7. Several cultures had superstitions that claimed that if a menstruating woman touched milk it would sour. Some also believed that if a menstruating woman touched meat it, too, would spoil.

8. In India, even today, Hindu women are not allowed to touch pickles or other delicacies when they are menstruating because it is thought that their touch could spoil the flavor.

9. Servants in India are not allowed to cook during their menstrual period because they might poison the food.

10. In a 1977 study conducted in the United States, 7 percent of adult respondents believed that a menstruating girl should be avoided by others.

11. In Bavaria it was believed that if a woman placed a few drops of her menstrual blood into a cop of coffee, the first man who drank it would marry her.

12. In several Native American traditions women who were having their menstrual periods were separated from the rest of the tribe and stayed in special huts called *kivas* until the period was over.

13. In some tribes women wore special face paint or bandages around their heads during their menstrual period. This was done to warn others.

14. Ancient warriors feared that if a menstruating woman came close to his sword, it would become instantly dulled.

15. Some Native American tribes killed a woman if she failed to tell her husband she was menstruating.

16. The ancient Persians would burn a man alive if he had sexual intercourse with a menstruating woman.

17. Some cultures believe that if a woman touches an animal during her period, the animal will die.

18. Many farmers believed that menstrual blood could create an evil influence on crops and weather.

19. Some farmers used menstrual blood as an insecticide.

20. Other farmers believed that if a menstruating woman touched a bud on a tree, it would wither within 24 hours.

21. It was once believed that if a woman looked in a mirror when she was menstruating, two round holes, corresponding to her eyes, would appear in the mirror.

22. Menstruating women were thought to be able to invoke a storm if they entered a boat.

23. In Northern France menstruating women were prohibited from visiting sugar refineries because men feared the sugar might turn black.

24. In Mexico, menstruating women were prohibited from visiting silver mines because men feared the ore might disappear.

25. Some cultures believed that menstruation first occurred when a serpent bit a woman.

26. Some tribes believed that girls began menstruating because they had had sexual intercourse with an ancestral spirit.

27. The term "red flag" comes from the tradition of women wearing a red bonnet around their heads to notify the tribe when they were having their menstrual period.

Heav'n has no rage like love to hatred turned,
nor hell a fury like a woman scorned.

—William Congreve

CHAPTER 2

Biology

Penis-Enlargement Methods That Work

1. Enlargement Surgery

Every year, over 6,000 American men have penis-enlargement surgery. There are two types of surgery: lengthening and widening. The average price is $4,000. One of the top enlargement surgeons in the country is Dr. Melvyn Rosenstein of Culver City, California. He has single-handedly performed over 2,000 enlargement surgeries. There is a debate among doctors as to the safety of these operations

Lengthening surgery. The lengthening surgery consists of cutting two ligaments connecting the penis to the pubic bone. Next, the penis is pulled forward from the body cavity. This operation adds around two inches to the length.

Widening surgery. Some men desire a thicker penis. The operation to achieve this goal is done by injecting fat under the skin of the penile shaft. The fat is taken from the lower abdomen and buttocks. The operation can double or triple the girth. The dangers are that the fat often melts away within a year and is reabsorbed by the body.

2. Penile Prosthesis

A penile prosthesis is an artificial rod or pump that is surgically placed inside the penis. Most doctors consider this to be the last resort for erectile problems. The rod version has the penis stay in a continual state of erection. Many men report this is useful, but it is much less popular than the pump because of safety and comfort issues.

3. Inflatable Implants

Surgeons perform approximately 20,000 inflatable-implant surgeries each year. The implant has three components: inflatable cylinders are placed inside the penis; tubing connects the cylinders to the abdomen; and the pump is placed in the scrotum. When a man pumps air into the cylinders they inflate and so does his penis.

The pressure-release valve connected to the pump reverses this process. Once again, the surgery is risky, expensive, and can be ineffective. However, it is rumored that comedian Flip Wilson had implant surgery.

4. Weight Loss

Weight loss is much more effective that you would ever think. For every 35 pounds of weight a man carries over his ideal weight his penis will appear to be one inch smaller. Overweight men tend to have fat covering the pubic bone at the base of the penis, with the result being that the penis appears smaller. Specialists recommend increasing exercise and decreasing fatty foods.

And the world's shrunken to a heap of hot flesh straining on a bed.

—E.R. Dodds

———◆———

Size Is Everything!: Animal Penis Lengths and Other Weird Penis Facts

We thought you might enjoy knowing the hard facts about the animal kingdom. The size of the penis greatly varies per animal. We have also included fascinating facts about animal penises and how they differ. For those who are grossed out by such things, skip this section.

1. *Humpback whales* have penises 10 feet long and 1 foot in diameter. Whales also emit the most amount of seminal discharge. They mate only once per year.

2. The class of animals known as *cetaceans*, which include dolphins and whales, have the largest penises among animals.

3. *Bottlenose dolphins* masturbate in unusual ways. They rub their penises on the backs of other males. When desperate, they masturbate on the back of a passing shark or turtle.

4. *Elephants* have 6 foot-long penises. Did you know that elephants masturbate using their trunks?

5. *Bulls* have penises 3 feet in length. The penises from dead bulls are often used as riding crops and whips.

6. *Stallions* have penises 2½ feet long.

7. A *rhinoceros* has a penis 2 feet in length.

8. Male *deer* masturbate by rubbing their antlers against tree trunks or on the ground. This produces both an erection and ejaculation.

9. The wonderful *pig* has an 18-inch penis. Their penises resemble corkscrews.

10. A *kangaroo* has a doubled-headed penis designed to match the double-horned vagina of the female.

11. The fierce *tiger* has an 11-inch penis. The male tiger masturbates using his paws.

12. The average *man* has a 6-inch penis.

13. The average *chimpanzee* has a 3-inch penis. They are able to perform fellatio on themselves.

14. *Platypus* are known for their 2¾-inch penises. Their penises have several pointed spines that point backwards (ouch).

15. The male *snowshoe hare's* penis turns white in the winter and is red during breeding season.

16. The *wild mallard* has a 1½-inch penis.

17. Male *orangutans* have penises around 1½ inches. They copulate while hanging upside down from trees.

18. The average *cat* has a 1-inch penis.

19. *Lizards* have two penises; one on each side of their bodies.

20. *Earthworms* are considered a hermaphrodite species. They have a penis and a vagina.

21. The *tapeworm* has over 22,000 different sex organs.

22. The small *bedbug* penis is curved and pointed.

23. *Mosquitoes* have tiny penises that measures 1/100 of an inch.

A stiff cock is nothing to be ashamed of.

—Linda Lovelace

---

7 Types of Birth Control

1. *The Pill*

The birth control pill is used by millions of women to prevent pregnancy. The pill contains estrogen and progesterone at higher than natural levels. This keeps the cervical mucus thick and thus difficult for sperm to get through. It also changes the uterus lining so that implantation of a fertilized egg is unlikely.

2. Norplant

Norplant® became available in 1990. It is an implant that is placed in a woman's arm. It comes in six rod-shaped capsules and lasts for five years. It is also the most effective form of birth control available today. The failure rate is 0.05 percent.

3. IUD

The intrauterine device (IUD) is a small plastic device that can also include metal or hormones. The IUD was first experimented with in the 1920s. It has one or two strings that hang down that help a woman to know if the device is in its proper place. A doctor inserts an IUD into a woman's uterus. IUDs are generally thought to be 98.4 percent effective. However, there was a sharp decline in use in the 1980s after many lawsuits were filed against manufacturers.

4. The Diaphragm

A diaphragm is a dome-shaped piece of thin rubber. The device is inserted into the vagina and fits snuggly over the cervix. A contraceptive jelly or cream is also applied to the diaphragm for maximum effectiveness. The diaphragm can be inserted into the vagina up to six hours before intercourse. The device works because it blocks sperm entering the entrance of the uterus. The sperm that remain in the vagina die after approximately eight hours. The failure rate is around 20 percent, although most failures are due to improper use.

5. Cervical Cap

The FDA approved the cervical cap in 1988. The cap works similarly to the diaphragm in that it fits over the cervix. It is a different shape, however. Like the diaphragm it is used with spermicidal cream or jelly. It can be left in for longer periods than can the diaphragm.

6. The Condom

We have mentioned the condom in several lists in this book. As you know, the condoms that are most effective are made from latex. (In the past, they were made from animal gut and other animal parts.) Condoms are not always a highly effective method of birth control because they are frequently put on and taken off incorrectly.

7. Spermicides

Spermicides take the form of contraceptive foams, creams, and jellies. They generally come in a tube or in a can along with a plastic applicator. The applicator is filled with spermicide, and the spermicide is inserted into the vagina before intercourse. It must be left in the vagina for at least six hours after intercourse.

Spermicide works by killing sperm. The inert base also helps by blocking the entrance to the cervix so sperm cannot enter. Spermicide is not a very effective method of birth control. Failure rate can be as high as 25 percent.

Alternative Birth Control Methods Still Being Tested

1. Male Hormone Methods

Tests are currently being run on men for a drug that will inhibit sperm production. In a recent research study hormone injections given to men inhibited sperm production by 98 percent.

2. Vaccines

A vaccine is also being developed for men that will use FSH or LHRH (luteinizing hormone releasing hormone). The LHRH works by shutting down the testes so that they cease producing sperm and testosterone. As a result, men taking the vaccine would have to take testosterone supplements. The FSH version has eliminated sperm production without impacting testosterone levels. FSH vaccines are currently being tested on monkeys.

3. Vaginal Rings

Researchers are currently developing a ring-shaped device that contains progesterone that will be inserted into the vagina and deliver progesterone to the body.

4. Sterilization

Do you want to never worry about getting pregnant, or getting someone pregnant again? Sterilization may be the way. Sterilization is a surgical procedure by which a man or woman is made incapable of reproduction. Some have confused this with castration, which sterilization is not. Sterilization is a popular method of birth control. Approximately 30 percent of married women are sterilized, and approximately 20 percent of married men.

> *Last night I discovered a new form of oral contraception—she said no.*
>
> —Woody Allen

————◆————

14 Physical Abnormalities and Anomalies in Men and Women

If you love *Ripley's Believe It or Not*, you will love this list. We've dug through the medical journals and texts from the past 125 years to find the absolute weirdest anomalies possible. By now you have probably grown to expect us to bring you the most bizarre and esoteric sex information available. This list will not let you down.

1. One odd penis abnormality is called *priapism*. This condition is when a man has an erection that will not go down. *Priapism* is quite dangerous because if the blood flow to the penis is restricted (like when it is continually erect), there is a high probability of nerve damage. In extreme cases the penis must be removed or amputated, or else blood clots can occur in various places around the body. Some men have this condition for weeks before damage occurs.

2. One of the oddest abnormalities for women is menstruation through the breasts. In the late 1800s there were several medical recordings of women menstruating through their nipples or other parts of their breasts. There is a recording from a London hospital in 1876 whereby a young woman was noted to menstruate monthly from her nipple and stomach. Women have also been known to menstruate through their eyes, ears, mouths, and other extremities.

3. Some men are known to have *polyorchids*, which means having more than two testicles. Many medical practitioners did not believe that this condition was real. However, in the *London Medical Record* of 1884 several British soldiers were said to have numerous testicles. In one instance the soldier had two testicles on one side and a third on the other side. The report claims that one man was seen by the coroner with six testicles.

4. In Scotland a woman was once noted by coroners to menstruate after she was dead. This was said to be caused by a high level of iron in her blood.

5. A traveling circus freak in England was rumored to have had the largest reported penis of all time. His name was "Mighty Mike," and he had a 25-inch phallus.

6. Several cases of unusual bladder conditions have been reported. Doctors who treated soldiers from the Battle of

McDowell, in Staunton, Virginia, in 1862, reported several cases of men noted to pass excrement through their urethra. In other cases men have been seen passing urine through their anus. Doctors also claim that there have been numerous cases in which excrement passed through a woman's vagina.

7. A male student at the University of Kentucky was said to be menstruating. He was part of a large number of men known to have menstrual periods. Men who are diagnosed with this condition are noted to have their "menstrual period" only on a very sporadic basis. Most men with this condition discharge blood through their urethra.

8. Enlarged clitorises have been seen for centuries. In 1824 a woman was seen by doctors in France with a five-inch clitoris. Her clitoris was so large that the woman at times could not have sex, as her clitoris was simply too large to allow a penis to enter. The largest clitoris on record was 12 inches in length.

9. In 1844 a boy who had two penises was seen by doctors. Each penis worked independently of the other; urine flowed from each. In another such case, the penises functioned at once; both urine and semen would be discharged at one time. There have been other occurrences of men with three and four penises.

10. In an 1891 annual medical meeting of doctors in the New York area, one of the topics of discussion was foreign items found in vaginas and how to conduct emergency medical procedures to remove such objects. They constructed a list of objects that they have had to remove. The list included glass, hairpins, beer mugs, bottles, sewing needles, compasses, a cork, and a pewter goblet. The group of doctors listed several items that are too disgusting even for this list.

11. In 1915 a surgeon wrote an article for *Allgem Medical Journal* that discussed various troubles and problems with semen. In the article the surgeon mentioned several unusual cases. One man was found to have black semen. The semen was thought to have passed by the bowel. Another hypothesis was that the semen included blood. Another article mentioned a man who had green semen. The cause was not known, and no hypothesis was given for potential causes.

12. In the 1800s several doctors reported cases of extremely short pregnancies. One women in Paris gave birth to a perfectly normal baby girl after only five months. Another reported case discusses a healthy baby girl born after four and a half months.

13. A rare penis medical disorder is called *micropenis*. When men have this condition their penis is abnormally small, usually less than two centimeters.

14. *Peyronie's disease* is a penis condition where the shaft becomes permanently bent at an angle. This condition makes urination and intercourse painful and difficult.

The borderline between normal and abnormal is by no means sharp, and there are all kinds of intermediate stages.

—J. Fabricius-Meller, *Sexual Life* (1944)

———◆———

How to Conduct a Testicular Examination

The American Cancer Society encourages all men to learn how to conduct a testicular self examination. It is thought to be best to give yourself the exam while in the shower or bath because the scrotum will be relaxed.

The 5 Steps to the Testicular Exam

1. Stand in front of the mirror and hold the penis out of the way of the testicles.

2. Examine each testicle separately. Hold it between the fingers and thumbs of each hand and gently roll it between the fingers.

3. Look and feel for any lumps or other masses of skin.

4. Look and feel for any changes in size, shape, or consistency.

5. If there are any problems contact your doctor immediately.

The Warning Signs of Testicular Cancer

1. There is an uncomfortable or painless lump in the testicle.

2. The testicle is enlarged or swollen.

3. There is aching or heaviness in the lower abdomen or in the scrotum.

A good sex life is not something you are born with, any more than you're born with the ability to cook, or crochet, or take shorthand.

Graham Masterson, *How to Drive Your Man Wild in Bed*

How to Conduct a Breast Self-Exam in 5 Minutes or Less

Breast cancer is one of the leading causes of death among women. It is very important for a woman to conduct self-exams for breast cancer on a regular basis because it could save her life. When breast cancer is found early, it can be treated, but if undetected for too long the results are then fatal.

The best time to conduct a breast self-exam is about one week after the menstrual period ends. At this time breasts are unlikely to be tender or swollen.

Steps to Conducting the Exam

1. Lie down with a pillow under the right shoulder and the right arm behind your head.

2. Use the middle three fingers to feel for lumps on the right breast. Press firmly to notice how the breast feels.

3. It is normal for there to be a firm ridge in the lower curve of each breast.

4. Feel the breast in an up and down, circular line. The manner is not so important. It is more important that you conduct the exam the same way everytime you do it.

5. Repeat steps one through four on the left breast.

6. Now stand up and place one arm behind your head.

7. Standing makes it easier to check the outer and the upper parts of your breasts, near your armpit. This area is where nearly half of all breast cancer is found.

8. If you notice changes or unusual swelling see your doctor at once.

*You know very well that love is, above all,
the gift of oneself!*

—Jean Anouilh, *Ardele* (1949)

———◆———

National Sex Information Hotlines

These phone lines are available for those who need them. They provide information, resources and counseling on several sexually related topics, and are all confidential and free.

1. *The San Francisco Sex Information Line: (415) 989-7374*
They will answer any sex-related questions.

2. *National STD Hotline: (800) 227-8922*
This hotline will provide you with answers about any sexually transmitted disease.

3. *National AIDS Hotline: (800) 342-2437*
This line will help find community resources for anyone who has HIV. They can also answer questions about HIV infection and prevention.

4. *Emergency Contraception Hotline: (888) NOT-2-LATE*
By calling this number you can immediately find the clinics and pharmacies nearest you that provide emergency contraception.

5. *Planned Parenthood: (800) 230-PLAN*
Planned Parenthood provides many services including contraception, counseling, STD referral, and sterilization. They can help you find a clinic near you.

6. Herpes Resource Center:

P.O. Box 13827; Research Triangle, NC 27709

The leading center on herpes information and support.

It's all this cold-hearted fucking that is death and idiocy.

—D.H. Lawrence

Abnormal Sex Organs and Abnormal Sex-Organ Development

Sex abnormalities are more common than you would think. They often occur before a child is born and require medical surgery. The cause is usually purely genetic, and researchers do not understand why they have continued to increase over time.

1. Turner's Syndrome

Very few girls are born with Turner's Syndrome. Turner's is when a girl is born with only one sex chromosome (X instead of XX). Girls appear female and show no other signs of the syndrome. However, girls with Turner's may not menstruate or develop breasts during adolescence. The treatment is usually female hormone therapy.

2. Klinefelter's Syndrome

Klinefelter's is similar to Turner's, but affects boys. Those with this syndrome have an extra X chromosome (XXY instead of XY). Some of the symptoms include smaller than normal testicles that produce minimal sperm, enlarged breasts, wider than normal hips, and a body type that has a female look to it. The current treatment is to include testosterone therapy with breast-reduction surgery.

3. Congenital Adrenal Hyperplasia (CAH)

This is very rarely found. CAH is caused by an overactive adrenal gland. As a result, female fetuses have an influx of male sex hormones and can be born with a penis and/or a scrotum. The treatment is usually hormone therapy and corrective surgery.

4. Hermaphroditism

Due to an imbalance of hormones in the mother's uterus during the development of the fetus, some babies are born with both male and female genitals. The treatment is usually a combination of surgery and hormonal therapy.

5. Intersex

Those who are considered intersex have a mixture of both male and female reproductive systems. At birth their gender is not clear. According to researchers such as John Money, those who are considered intersex can be classified as either gender as long as the classification occurs before they reach 18 months, the requisite surgeries are completed, and hormonal therapy is administered. However, some intersexual adults feel the gender choice made for them in infancy was not correct.

6. 5-α Reductase Syndrome

This syndrome is similar to CAH, but more uncommon. It was first noted and studied in 1974 in the Dominican Republic. The syndrome occurs due to a genetic endocrine problem, whereby males appear to be female at birth, and are born with a vagina instead of a scrotum and have a clitoris-sized penis. While they are genetically male, they are treated as and appear to be female. At puberty they spontaneously develop a penis.

The reproduction of mankind is a great marvel and mystery. Had God consulted me in the matter, I should have advised him to continue the generation of the species by fashioning them of clay.

—Martin Luther (Sixteenth Century)

———◆———

Mating Habits of Animals

We can learn about our own mating habits by exploring the animal kingdom. As you read these examples of animal copulation, you just might notice that many of them are not too far from the ways in which humans mate. It is pretty scary to see that we are not as sophisticated as we think.

1. *Bulls* do not have much of a sex life. They copulate in one thrust. The entire act takes less than 20 seconds.

2. The *hummingbird* family are the smallest birds in the world. Most have bodies approximately two inches in length. Their mating rituals involve several males competing for the opportunity to mate with a female. The males attempt to win over the female by performing stunts in the air, each bird trying to outdo the others. The female watches from a branch. After each male has had a chance to impress the female, she picks one. The winner immediately copulates with the female while the others watch with envy.

3. *Scorpions* are odd creatures. When they copulate these normally antisocial creatures begin by being quite kind toward one another. Their mating starts with soft caresses and dancing. They stand on their heads and intertwine their tails into

a lovers knot and then stroke each other's body. They then rear up on their hind legs and begin dancing. This sexually stimulates both partners and inspires them to find a private place to copulate. However, in the morning only the female survives. She kills the male after the hot sex session.

4. The male *rat* likes a challenge. He ejaculates nearly twice as much sperm when he mates with a female who has recently been with other males.

5. The sex world of the *octopus* can be quite bizarre. They start out in a romantic manner with the male massaging the female with one of his eight arms. The massage has a stimulating quality for both of them. At some point the massage intensifies and the color of their bodies change, indicating they are ready for copulation. The male then removes several "containers" of semen from a warehouse in one of his tentacles. He then inserts his penis into the female's mantle cavity. In the best of all worlds his sperm then swells and bursts, thus fertilizing the eggs. However, as the male maneuvers his penis, he blocks the female's oxygen flow. This can cause her to be greatly aroused or to resist him. There have been cases of the female ripping the man's sexual organ off his body during the mating. As you've probably guessed, this is not a good thing.

6. *Sage grouse* have sex only one night per year. And during that evening they have sex 100 times. That's a lot of sex in one night.

7. The *African blood fluke* is an unusual parasitic worm. They copulate by having the female crawl inside the male's body. She then moves to his pelvic region where she lays her eggs. The eggs are then flushed out of his body into a river where they hatch.

8. *Lions* are known to copulate frequently; one study showed a lion copulating 86 times in one day.

9. The *cockroach* is said to be one of the more intelligent insects. There are over 3,500 known types of cockroaches. In one of the most popular species, the couple begin mating while facing each other. Next, they start rubbing antennae. The male quickly becomes aroused from this activity. He then raises his wings, and the female mounts him. As she mounts one of his penises hooks onto her body. The male then turns around again so that they are tail to tail. His remaining penises all lock into place, and they copulate for at least two hours.

10. The female *bedbug* has no vagina and so the male must rip open her stomach with his penis to deposit his sperm into her.

11. The male *mink* is known for his high libido. Mating rituals between minks tend to be quite savage. The male constantly attacks the female, and she continuously repels him. They continue this process several times until the male overtakes the female. They copulate in such a rough manner because the female doesn't release her ripe eggs until they are both in a state of extreme excitation.

12. The male *mosquito* rips open the female pupae with his penis in order to copulate. The female often dies during this process.

13. The *praying mantis* is known for its brutal behavior, but it might be worse than you thought. When they mate the female approaches the male. After the male knows she is interested in him, he accepts her advances. So then what happens? The female literally bites off his head. But does the male mantis stop? No, he is still full of sex drive. His better half then mounts her, they continue getting it on, and then finally he falls to the ground dead. The next step for the female is to eat the rest of his body.

14. The *callicecus monkey* mates for life. After mating for the first time they begin marking their territory and guard it for the rest of their lives.

15. *Bats* have sex upside down. This is no surprise; however, the details are not usually discussed. When they mate the female grips onto the ceiling while the male grips the female from below, gripping her body and pushing his belly against her spine. His penis is long and angled so that this type of copulation is effective.

16. The *crocodile* is one of the harshest creatures when it comes to mating rituals. When the male is excited he finds the first female he can and basically attacks her. He roars loudly and opens his jaws. The male quickly overpowers the female and throws her on her back. He pins her down and pushes himself into her while she lies on her back. The entire ritual usually takes less than eight minutes.

17. *Bonobo chimps* are one of the horniest species of animals on the face of the planet. They have sex on average every 90 minutes, each sex act lasting for around 13 seconds. They have sex when they make friends, when they mate, when they play, and even before they eat. They even have a practice that looks like French kissing. And they engage in oral sex. Females are the dominant sex in the Bonobo world, and lesbian sex is prevalent. This species is known, however, to be one of the most peaceful animal species. Most conflicts are resolved through . . . sex.

There's nothing that is as passionate as when you are at the end of each other's rope. It is such an amazing feeling. You feel most alive when you're closest to death.

—Brad Pitt

Penis-Enlargement Techniques and Machines That Do Not Work

1. Kama Sutra

The *Kama Sutra* offered one bizarre method to enlarge the penis. The technique is done by rubbing the penis with tepid water. Next, rub the penis with a solution of honey and ginger. This technique was to be done daily for three months and claimed to add inches to the penis.

2. The Penis Stretch/Super Stretch

This "device" has been advertised since the 1970s. While it sound very impressive, it is nothing more than a rubber band used to pull the shaft of the penis in a downward motion. This device has been called dangerous by several doctors, and its method, to be worn by a man during his daily activities, has shown to do nothing but rupture nerve endings and cause unnecessary pain and discomfort.

3. Use of Bells

In the country of Myanmar metal bells have been used for centuries for penis rituals. Several tribes in this country implant small metal bells under their foreskins. They claim that the bells increase the girth of the penis and are an added turn-on for women. Plus the bells ring during intercourse for added mood music. This procedure is not currently done in the United States, but surely a piercing shop somewhere might attempt this technique for you.

4. Penis Pumps

Before Viagra,® doctors frequently prescribed these devices (technically called hypermiators) to men who had a difficult time maintaining erections. Pumps were fairly effective in helping with impotence and erectile dysfunction. There has been little or no evidence that these devices enlarge a man's penis in any permanent fashion. Some of these devices are battery operated, some are plugged into the wall. Either way, none works for penis enlargement.

5. Arabian Tinctures

Ready for some of the most bizarre techniques of all times? Some Arab traditions claimed that by attaching bruised leeches to the penis the skin would somehow expand and increase in size. They also claimed that penises from boiled asses could be used to rub over the shaft to help inspire growth. Do not try this at home!

6. Weights

Some men have selected to use weights, which hang from the penis, as an enlargement method. This method has been used in primitive cultures for several centuries. While it is painful and dangerous, it has not been shown to work.

7. Roman Traditions

In Imperial Rome many men would insert golden rings, coins, and charms into their foreskin. This ritual was said to have the penis appear to be longer and to increase the sexual pleasure of a woman during intercourse.

> *Take every pain in infancy to enlarge the privy member of boys (by massage and the application of stimulants), since a well-grown specimen never comes amiss.*
>
> —Gabriello Fallopio, *Obseruationes Anotomicae* (1561)

———◆———

13 Biological Facts About Men

1. Thirty-three percent of men between the ages of 30 and 40 have begun balding.

2. Sixty-five percent of men have wavy hair.

3. It is estimated that a man will grow 27.5 feet of facial hair during his lifetime.

4. The average man is 5 foot 9.

5. The average male thigh is 21 inches.

6. Ten percent of men have curly hair.

7. Six percent of American men have red hair.

8. Forty-four percent of men wear glasses.

9. Ten percent of all men have black hair.

10. By the age of 100 there are only 18 men per 100 women.

11. Men, on average, weight 172 pounds.

12. Men's life expectancy is seven years less than women's.

13. Men suffer more mental illnesses than women.

You never know a man until you know how he loves.

—Sigmund Freud

13 Biological Facts About Women

Yes, it is true, we do not understand women at all. There are various facts that most men choose to ignore or deny. Biological facts, however, never lie.

1. The average woman has 400,000 ova.

2. The average woman is 5 foot 3 inches tall.

3. Ten percent of American women have curly hair.

4. The typical American woman wears a 36B bra.

5. Fifty-four percent of women wear glasses.

6. The average thickness of a hymen is between .05 and .10 inches.

7. The average clitoris is one inch long.

8. Fifteen percent of American woman have blond hair.

9. The average woman weighs 143 pounds.

10. One out of every thousand women are born without a uterus.

11. A female egg is 1/175 of an inch wide.

12. Women have 75 percent more scent glands than men.

13. The pH level of an average vagina is 4.0 to 5.0, which rates as fairly acidic.

I've always thought it's the role of women to spread sex and sunshine in the lives of men.

—Jayne Mansfield

15 Body-Language Signals That Show a Woman Is Interested in a Man

Some people swear by body-language signals. Body-language signals are difficult to teach and when applied in the real world can be confusing. We thought you should know some of the common body-language signs, however, so you can determine if they really do work. Here are some common signs that a woman is interested in a man.

1. Dilated pupils

2. Swollen lips

3. Flips hair

4. Twirls hair

5. Flips eyelids

6. Smiles

7. Licks lips

8. Gives sidelong glances

9. Holds gaze

10. Looks at you and then quickly looks away

11. Changes posture to alert stance

12. Turns body toward you

13. Tilts head toward you

14. Touches you

15. Dangles shoe

The first kiss is magic, the second intimate, the third routine. After that you just take the girl's clothes off.

—Raymond Chandler

———◆———

11 Stages of Male Orgasm

Researchers have been able to figure out the distinct stages of a male orgasm. They have found 11 separate stages that occur rapidly during the orgasm process. Yet, the male orgasm usually lasts only seconds. We have provided this information for you to use.

Stage 1: The penis shaft reaches its maximum width, rigidity, and length.

Stage 2: The penis head, technically called the glans, darkens and swells due to vasocongestion of blood.

Stage 3: The Cowper's glands moisten the tip of the penis. The tip also widens.

Stage 4: The testes rise and rotate, thus coming into closer contact with the man's body. The testes also increase in size by 50 to 100 percent.

Stage 5: Blood pressure rises.

Stage 6: The heart rate shoots from 70 beats per minute to over 150, sometimes as high as 180.

Stage 7: Breathing becomes shallow and rapid. Breathing rate increases by nearly three times the normal rate.

Stage 8: Muscles tighten. Facial muscles tighten, as do the toes, feet, and hands. Sometimes the man emits cries through his vocal cords.

Stage 9: The nipples harden and swell. Some men find that their nipples become tender and very sensitive.

Stage 10: Blood rushes throughout the body, causing the skin in the face and chest to appear more red than usual.

Stage 11: After orgasm many men break out with sweat on their palms and feet.

A man must be potent and orgasmic to ensure the future of the race. A woman only needs to be available.

—Masters and Johnson

———◆———

14 Bizarre Aphrodisiacs

While some aphrodisiacs may seem strange, there may be a modicum of factual evidence backing up claims that they do indeed work. Some methods have been shown to increase sex drive, testosterone, and so forth, but many of the outrageous claims for aphrodisiacs simply go too far. We have assembled a list of a few of the most bizarre aphrodisiacs you can make sure *not* to use.

1. Lizard Flesh
This strange substance is known to drive anyone crazy with lust and have them jump your bones immediately. The problem is that you first have to skin a lizard and then eat the flesh. Simply put, this is no more than an outrageous claim that seems too

bizarre, even to us. Lizard became a popular amorous substance in Arab countries where it was served with wine and powdered with sugar.

2. Lion's Fat

The fat from a lion was a popular aphrodisiac in Medieval times. It was said that the fat had to be procured in a ritual manner. The fat was then cooked over a fire and consumed in the dead of night. We do not recommend that you go to your local zoo and kill a lion to try this at home.

3. Peas

According to the infamous book *The Perfumed Garden,* a mixture of peas, onions, cinnamon, ginger, and cardamom is a perfect way to create passion in yourself and others. No one else will corroborate this claim.

4. Pork

For the meat lover in you, pork may be one of the best ways to become aroused and rejuvenate your love life. Some claim that a dish mixed with pork and milk can rejuvenate one's love life. Though pork is obviously not kosher, some swear by it.

5. Rocket Salad

According to the Roman poet Ovid, a salad containing olive oil, vinegar, pepper, and chopped garlic will inspire amorous desire in anyone who feasts on it. The men we know can't get a date when they've got garlic breath. How did Ovid do it?

6. Animal Genitalia

Some cultures believed that eating the testicles of an animal would dramatically raise the testosterone level of the man eating the animal parts. This method was particularly popular among Frenchmen and their horses.

7. Ants

One popular Medieval recipe calls for dried black ants. They were to be killed by pouring hot oil over them and then they were stored in glass jars ready for quick use. Hmm, ants and sex . . .

8. Human Blood

During Roman times some believed that human blood contained the power to inspire great lust in women. Many men would cut themselves and drip their blood into food fed to women or into liqueurs served to women. In a recent experiment carried out by Louis and Copeland, we tried it and the women slapped us.

9. Brains

In some Mediterranean countries the brain from a sheep, a calf, or a pig is served for its erotic effects. They are known as a delicacy and a powerful sexual stimulant. Some cultures even believe that dove brains are a sexual stimulant. We'll put it to you this way: it takes brains not to eat brains.

10. Human Corpse

A very unusual belief from the Hindu tradition is to create a mixture of part burnt human flesh, part Indian plant *vatodbhranta*, and part powdered bones from a peacock. The mixture is then diluted with water and applied to the penis. It then is said to result in sexual dominance. If you have access to burnt human flesh, do not tell us about it. The powdered peacock bones are strange enough.

11. Crocodile

Several South American traditions involve the use of a crocodile to inspire sexual performance. Some believed that by eating the tail of a young crocodile a man would be able to have unlimited sexual power, while others believed that a mixture of crocodile excrement and honey rubbed onto the penis would create everlasting sexual power. No comment.

12. Kidneys

Along with brains, kidneys are said to be quite powerful sexual stimulants. Some cultures believe that eating kidneys from sheep, pigs, or cattle would improve the sexual stamina of any man. Yeah, right.

13. Lard

Lard isn't just for cooking. Lard mixed with garlic has also been used as a stimulant when rubbed on a flaccid penis. Please do not try this at home. If you are a man who is married or in a committed relationship, do not even tell your woman you read about the power of lard.

14. Fish Exposure

In the Middle Ages one popular method for increasing male sex drive was to place a fish into a woman's vagina until it died. Then the fish was cooked and served to the man. Ladies, we know you constantly sacrifice to make your relationships work, but this is simply going to far.

Healthy, lusty sex is wonderful.

—John Wayne

Birth Control Methods That Do Not Work

There are several popular methods used for birth control that simply do not work. People tend to use these methods and ignore all the research that shows the inconsistencies and potential risks. We strongly suggest that you use proven methods if you are truly concerned about pregnancy risks and STD risks. Here is the list of birth control methods not to try:

1. Douching

Some people believe that douching can be an effective birth control method. They are wrong. The theory is that an acidic solution inserted into the vagina can kill sperm. While this is true, sperm need only seconds to swim into the uterus. As a result, douching does not reach the sperm.

2. Withdrawal Method

Women who actually trust a man to withdraw before spraying his sperm inside them are pretty gullible. While this method is one of the most ancient forms of birth control and is still used today throughout the world, it is not effective.

Failure can happen for a variety of reasons. A man's "pre-come" contains sperm and thus can easily impregnate the woman. A man can also ejaculate near a woman's vagina and accidentally penetrate her with sperm. A man can also lose control of himself and ejaculate before he has the willpower to withdraw. As you can see, this method is real trouble.

3. Rhythm Method

This is the only form of birth control to be officially approved by the Roman Catholic Church. The theory is that if a couple abstains from sex during a woman's fertility period, then she will not become pregnant.

Forms of the rhythm method include:

a. Calendar Method

Some couples use the calendar method. It is based on the assumption that ovulation occurs approximately 14 days before the start of menstruation. This method works best for women who have a reliable 28-day cycle. This means that a woman ovulates on day 14, or at least on day 13 or 15. Women who are not reliable can keep notes on their cycle for six months and thus determine their shortest cycle and longest cycle. They can then use this method to figure out which days of the month she must be abstinent.

b. Basal Temperature Method

The basal method is more accurate than the calendar method, but is still not advised. When following this method, a woman takes her temperature daily upon waking. Her temperature will remain at a consistently low level during her preovulatory phase. It is said that the day of ovulation her temperature will drop, and then the day after ovulation her temperature will slightly rise. Her temperature will then stay at the higher temperature for the remainder of her cycle. It is assumed that it is safe to have sex three days after ovulation. One of the problems with this method is that women's temperatures can fluctuate for reasons other than ovulation. Furthermore, this method greatly limits the number of days the woman can have sex.

c. Cervical Mucus Method

This method looks at the variations in the mucus produced by the cervix during a woman's cycle. This method assumes that it is relatively safe to have sex a few days after menstruation. In this time period no mucus is produced and there is a sense of dryness in the vagina. The next period is that there are several days of mucus discharge in the middle of a cycle. The start of a cycle is a time when the mucus is white or cloudy. The amount of mucus increases and the mucus becomes clearer. This is followed by peak days when the mucus is like a raw egg white and the vagina is highly lubricated. Ovulation then occurs within 24 hours. A woman can determine that she must refrain from sex from the first day of mucus discharge until four days after the peak days. After that, she is said to be able to have as much sex as she wants. This method is very hard to track and hard to determine. There is a very low success rate.

d. Sympto-thermal Method

This method employs two of the other rhythm methods. Usually a woman will use the calendar method and the mucus method to increase the success of tracking her cycle.

*It is now quite lawful for a Catholic woman
to avoid pregnancy by resorting to mathematics,
though she is still forbidden to resort
to physics or chemistry.*

—H. L. Mencken

---◆---

19 Fun Facts About the Penis and Scrotum

1. The origin of the word "penis" comes from Latin, meaning "tail."

2. Men live longer without testicles. Men who are castrated have a life expectance of 13 years longer than do men with testicles.

3. The average penis is six inches long when erect.

4. The average male ejaculates approximately 18 quarts of sperm in his lifetime.

5. The men in one Australian tribe shake penises instead of hands when greeting each other.

6. The left testicle on most men hangs lower than the right.

7. The average man achieves an erection in less than ten seconds.

8. In one ejaculation there can be more than 600 million sperm.

9. An average man can ejaculate his semen nearly two feet.

10. Aristotle thought that small penises were better for conception than larger ones. He thought that since the penis was smaller, the sperm had less distance to travel.

11. Sperm count in men continues to decline each year they age.

12. The average teaspoon of semen contains five calories.

13. Penile cancer accounts for 1.5 percent of all cancers contracted by men.

14. The average sperm is four microns long (there are 1,000 microns per millimeter).

15. Masters and Johnson note that three men per 1,000 can perform self-fellatio.

16. In the Middle Ages it was thought that men and women produced equal amounts of sperm.

17. The average testicle is two inches long and one inch in breadth.

18. The average orgasm for men lasts between three and ten seconds.

19. On an annual basis, a typical man will produce billions of sperm.

Don't forget, the penis is mightier than the sword.

—Jay Hawkins

A Taste of Latex! 5 Latex Items Used During Sex

Latex is the way. Fetish fashion models wear latex sex outfits, and nearly everyone has experienced a latex condom at least once in their lives. The best part is that latex has proven to be effective in protecting everyone from the risks of bodily fluid exchange. Latex can become a fun part of any sex routine. Note: Latex should be used only with water-based lubricants. Lubricants that are oil-based can break down the rubber in latex and cause a condom to be useless.

Here is the list of latex products available for use in your bedroom tonight:

1. Condoms
Latex condoms are the only type that protect both parties from HIV and other diseases. Available in most drug stores and the bathrooms in your finer truck stops.

2. Dental Dams
Dental dams usually come in six-inch squares of latex. They are used by dentists during oral surgery. They can also be used as an effective way to protect persons while engaging in oral sex. Many couples have found that dental dams can add to the pleasure of an oral sex experience. It is recommended that dental dams be thrown away after use. Dental dams are available in a variety of colors and flavors (from bubble gum to vanilla).

3. Latex Face Mask
Along with dental dams, the latex face mask can be worn to protect the one who is giving oral stimulation to a partner. These masks are worn over the mouth and are designed to make it easier to give oral sex. Some folks even wear face masks because they are turned on by how they look.

4. Latex Gloves

Ready to really play doctor? This cheap sex tool can be used to protect fingers and hands from contacting mucous membranes. They can also be used to give a hand job to your lover. You can even use gloves in an anal or vaginal fisting contest. Gloves should not be reused.

5. Finger Cots

No, we are not talking about sleeping on a bed of fingers. These items are similar to small condoms that can be placed on a finger. Finger cots are effective for sex involving anal stimulation or finger penetration—pretty much any sexual activity involving fingers being inserted or stuck into any bodily area. Finger cots can also be used to protect butt plugs, small dildos, and vibrators.

Make war, not love. It's safer.

—Henny Youngman

———◆———

Strange and Unusual Orgasms

There can be back of the neck orgasms, bottom of the foot orgasms, and palm of the hand orgasms.

—Masters and Johnson

———◆———

Yes, there are many strange types of orgasms. Some people have spontaneous orgasms while other people have orgasms from things you would never believe. Here is a list of some of the most bizarre.

1. A woman in Milwaukee was said to have a spontaneous orgasm from a bump to her head. She was playing bingo and accidentally bumped her head against the scoreboard, causing an orgasm.

2. Some women have reported having orgasms from kissing.

3. Many women have experienced orgasms from having their nipples touched, sucked, and so on.

4. Some women can have orgasms from merely thinking sexual thoughts.

5. One woman was rumored to have an orgasm from driving over 100 mph on the highway.

6. We read one account of a woman spontaneously having an orgasm because she was nervous about an exam. The nervousness caused the orgasm.

7. Some men can have orgasm while bringing a woman to orgasm.

8. At Rutgers University a professor researched women who claimed to be able to have "psychic orgasms." These orgasms occur from sexual fantasy. The research showed that there was no physiological difference between a "psychic orgasm" and a regular one.

9. Some women can have orgasms when they hear a sexy male voice.

10. Several dominatrixes claim that they can train men to orgasm on command.

11. Prostitutes in ancient times claimed that they could bring a man to orgasm by tugging on his pubic hair.

12. Many men report orgasms from receiving anal sex.

13. Some women report experiencing orgasms from being spanked.

14. Many women can experience orgasms while urinating.

At the moment of climax there is oneness with you and your husband and with God . . . When you come together, it's like the church is brought up to meet Christ in the air.

—Anita Bryant

———◆———

Men's Sexual Frequency as They Age

Men do keep having sex as they age, but as you can see, the frequency of sex goes down . . . while 12 percent of men aged 18 to 24 have sex four or more times a week, by the time they reach 50, only 3 percent of them are. Still, the numbers aren't *that* bad . . .

Age	Never	Few Times/ Year	Few Times/ Month	2–3 Times/ Week	4+/ Week
18–24	15%	21%	24%	28%	12%
25–29	7	15	31	36	11
30–39	8	15	37	33	6
40–49	9	18	40	27	6
50–59	11	22	43	20	3

According to Sex in America survey, University of Chicago, 1994

Sex after ninety is like trying to shoot pool with a rope. Even putting my cigar in its holder is a thrill.

—George Burns

———◆———

Tips for Using a Condom

Condoms have a long, long history. A French cave painting of a man wearing a primitive condom indicates they've been around for more than 3,000 years. About that same time, men in Egypt wore condoms as a sign of rank. Now they are mostly just worn during sex.

A federally funded study found that 0.66 percent of condoms tested (more than 1 in 200) failed. The failures happened in three ways:

1. Allowing water or air to escape

2. Failing air-burst tests

3. Leaking HIV virus

So condoms do sometimes fail. Here's a list of ways to help prevent failures in your own experience:

1. Be sure to use plenty of lubrication. Condoms sometimes tear, and it's often because of lack of lubrication.

2. Make sure your condom is the right size. Condoms come in narrow, large, and huge, and it's important to know which size they are. We knew a man who hated condoms for years because they were so tight—it turned out he was using condoms that were too small. A too-small condom is more likely to tear, a too-large one to slide off.

3. Notice which way the condom is rolled, and be sure to roll it the right way when you are putting it on the penis. Trying to unroll it the wrong way can really ruin the moment, or even the condom.

4. Squeeze the tip of reservoir condoms to keep air out when you put it on.

5. Hold the base of the condom when withdrawing to avoid leaking.

6. Withdraw before the penis is completely soft, to avoid leaking.

7. Don't reuse condoms.

8. Use condoms on sex toys to keep them clean, or on any toy that gets inserted in more than one person. Change the condom before moving any toy from one person to another.

Whenever I hear people discussing birth control,
I always remember that I was the fifth.

—Clarence Darrow

———◆———

Reasons Not to Circumcise Your Son

Circumcision became routine in the United States in the late 1800s, when doctors claimed it would reduce masturbation and that it was more hygienic. Here are some reasons to not circumcise your son:

1. Sensitivity is reduced. Circumcision basically makes an internal organ—the glans at the end of the penis—into an external one. The once-covered glans of the penis become toughened and "cornified," thus losing sensitivity (a commonly quoted figure is up to 40 percent of sensitivity lost).

2. According to the National Center of Health Statistics, in the 1980s, 90 percent of American baby boys were circumcised.

3. In the 1990s, that number of circumcised boys fell to 59 percent.

4. Most circumcisions on baby boys are performed without anesthetic. One study found that boys who were circumcised without anesthetic were more sensitive and reactive to pain during later vaccinations than were boys who were circumcised using anesthetic. Uncircumcised boys showed the least pain response of all.

5. Circumcising baby boys can result in a condition called *meatal stenosis*. This is an inflammation or ulceration of the meatus (the urinary opening). The foreskin covers the opening of the urethra and protects it from urine or feces. Without the foreskin, meatal stenosis can occur, though it rarely occurs in uncircumcised babies.

6. A small number of circumcised men don't experience desensitization—they experience hypersensitive irritation when the glans of their penis rubs against anything, such as clothing.

7. Circumcision can leave too little skin for the penis to "grow into." After all, an infant is going to get a lot bigger. Apparently, erections can be uncomfortable for an adult male if too little skin is left during circumcision.

> *My brain is my second favorite organ.*
>
> —Woody Allen

Reasons to Circumcise Your Son

Then there's the other side. . . . Plenty of people still think male circumcision is a really bright idea:

1. One study showed that uncircumcised infants have a ten times greater risk of urinary tract infections.

2. Another researcher found that the intact foreskin is a good growth area for bacteria that can travel up the urethra and cause kidney infections.

3. Circumcision may help prevent a cancer called *penile carcinoma*. There are approximately 1,000 cases of penile carcinoma in the United States each year.

4. The moist skin under the foreskin is more easily penetrated by bacteria and infectious agents than the more "cornified" skin of a circumcised penis.

5. Uncircumcised males may experience *phimosis*, an inability to retract the foreskin, making it difficult or impossible to urinate.

6. Uncircumcised males may also experience *paraphimosis*, a painful condition in which the foreskin can be retracted but not brought back forward again.

7. A foreskin can become inflamed in a condition called *posthitis*.

8. An uncircumcised boy may experience embarrassment in the locker room, if the look of his penis doesn't conform to those of other boys.

The genitals themselves have not undergone the development of the rest of the human form in the direction of beauty.

—Sigmund Freud

Surgical Foreskin Restoration Techniques

What is *foreskin restoration?* Some men who believe they have lost significant sensitivity in their penises have the foreskin restored. There are two approaches to this: surgical and do-it-yourself. Here's a list of the surgical methods:

1. **Surgical platinum ring implant.** A platinum ring is implanted under the skin of the penile shaft, drawn forward over the glans, and tightened so it can't slip back. In time this apparently stretches the skin so that at least, a partial, foreskin is created. There are problems, though. When the ring is removed, there may not be as much skin over the glans as hoped, and a ring of fibrous tissue can form around the platinum ring, which may also have to be removed surgically. Also, this procedure is best for men who were circumcised in such a way as to have enough loose skin for this procedure. Most American-style circumcisions are too "tightly done" for this to work.

2. **Prepuce reconstruction by granulation tissue.** When the edges of a wound are kept pulled apart, scar tissue forms between them—this process is known as granulation. By cutting a circle along the penile shaft, the edges pulled slightly apart and allowed to heal, a little more skin is grown. If this is done about a dozen times over a several-year period, enough tissue to cover the glans can be created. Kids, don't try this at home.

3. **Scrotal graft technique.** This technique requires multiple surgeries and up to eight months to heal. Briefly put, an incision is made around the shaft of the penis an inch or so above the glans, and this skin is pulled forward to cover the glans. The (now terribly naked) penis is then surgically put straight down into an opening in the scrotal sac to heal (the very tip of the penis protruding from a slit in the bottom). After this

has all healed (months and months) the scrotal skin is slit to release the now healed, foreskinned penis. Even writing about this makes us shudder.

4. **Z-plasty technique.** This approach does create more skin to go forward over the glans, but you trade circumference of skin around the penile shaft for this new length. And it's just skin length—this isn't a way to enlarge your penis. Basically, three Z-shaped incisions are made along the length of the penis, which are realigned and sutured to create more length but less girth in the penis. These surgical realignments can create a partially restored foreskin.

5. **Skin grafting procedures (free-grafting).** Skin is taken from somewhere else in the body and grafted into a new foreskin. Once again, it's a series of surgeries, and, once again, it can produce mixed results. Skin colors may not match, there may be hair on the newly transplanted skin. And, of course, you have to give up skin that you were using someplace else.

*When they circumcised Herbert they threw away
the wrong bit.*

—Lloyd George

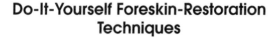

Do-It-Yourself Foreskin-Restoration Techniques

Okay, so the surgical foreskin-restoration techniques all sound a little scary and *very* painful and intrusive. Why not opt for doing it yourself? Satisfied users say that this technique does work to restore the foreskin (and thus increase the sensitivity of the glans and improve sex!), if you are willing to follow all the steps. (*Note:* Don't follow the instructions that we have here—get all the specific details from one of the resources we list, and do the program with the knowledge and supervision of an open-minded doctor.)

In brief, however, the steps are these:

1. Use tape to pull as much skin as you can over the head of the penis, and hold it there.

2. If you were loosely circumcised, you can, alternatively, pull the skin completely over the glans, and hold it there with a ring of tape.

3. After a few months of doing this daily, you may be stretched enough to begin to tape small weights to the developing foreskin to continue pulling the skin forward.

4. At this stage some men make a small foam cone that fits over the head of the penis for the newly developing foreskin to grow along. This is to create greater length. A man may use a series of increasingly larger cones as he creates a long-enough foreskin.

5. Though the program may seem unusual, it shouldn't be painful, change skin color, or apply too much pressure.

Man is in the wrong in being ashamed to exhibit it . . . when he ought to adorn and display it.

—Leonardo da Vinci

Resources for Helping You (or a Loved One!) Create a New Foreskin

If you want to create a new foreskin for yourself, you'll need more information about doing it. Try these resources:

1. *The Joy of Uncircumcising! Restore Your Birthright and Maximize Sexual Pleasure.* Jim Bigelow, Ph.D.

2. *Decircumcision: Circumcision Practices and Foreskin Restoration Methods*, Gary M. Griffin, MBA

3. The National Organization of Circumcision Information Resource Centers (NOCIRC), P.O. Box 2512, San Anselmo, CA 94979-2512. (415) 488-9883. Fax: (415) 488-9660. http://www.nocirc.org

4. National Organization of Restoring Men (NORM) 3205 Northwood Drive #209, Concord, CA 94520-4506. (510) 827-4077. Fax: (510) 827-4119. http://www.norm.org

5. National Organization to Halt the Abuse and Routine Mutilation of Males (NOHARMM), 460795, San Francisco, CA 94146. (415) 826-9351. Fax: (305) 768-5967. http://www.noharmm.org

6. Uncircumcising Information and Resources Center (UNCIRC), (408) 375-4326

7. Doctors Opposing Circumcision (D.O.C.), 2442 NW Market St #42, Seattle, WA 98107. (206) 368-8358. Fax:(206) 368-9428. http://faculty.washington.edu/gcd/DOC/

8. Nurses for the Rights of the Child (NRC), 369 Montezuma #354, Santa Fe, NM 87501. (505) 989-7377. http://www.cirp.org/nrc/

9. Circumcision Resource Center (CRC), (617) 523-0088. http://
www.circumcision.org

*In the United States, about 1,325,000 neo-natal
circumcisions are performed each year.
The practice gives cause for alarm, since
it results in about 230 deaths each year
as a result of accident or infection.*

—Roy Eskapa

◆

Types of Female Circumcision

The term "female circumcision," by the way, is a misnomer—only
one type of circumcision preformed on women is anything at all
like what is routinely performed on men. A more proper term
would be "severe female genital mutilation," as some of these procedures remove the full clitoris and the inner and outer labia of
the vagina. The circumcision men experience cannot hold a candle to the brutality and severity of the more brutal types of "circumcisions" performed on women. The World Health Organization
estimates that over 80 million women in Africa have been circumcised—it is not known what percentage of these women have the
least severe of these mutilations, similar to male circumcision—or
the most severe of these mutilations.While the origins of female
circumcision are unknown, as long ago as the fifth century B.C. it
was practiced by the Phoenicians, Hittites, Ethiopians, and
Egyptians. Today the procedure is usually performed under unhy-
gienic conditions by an elderly woman (an *ouddo* in Somalia, *daya*
in Egypt, *khafedha* in Sudan) usually as part of an adolescent girl's

initiation into adulthood. It is done without anesthetic, often with a razor blade or other sharp implement.

Here are the types of female circumcision. Be warned—this is not for the faint of heart:

1. **Sunnah:** This is the least invasive of the types of female circumcision, and is most like the circumcision routinely experienced by men in the West. This is the removal of the prepuce of the clitoris—not the removal of the clitoris itself.

2. **Clitoridectomy:** This is the total removal of the clitoris. The clitoris is punctured, then rubbed to expose it, then cut off.

3. **Excision:** This is the removal of the clitoris and the labia minora.

4. **Intermediate:** This is the removal of the clitoris, the labia minora, and sometimes part of the labia majora.

5. **Infibulation** (also called Pharaonic circumcision): This is the removal of the clitoris, the labia minora, some of the labia majora, and sewing together the two sides of the vulva, leaving only a small opening for menstrual fluid and urine. The wound is usually held closed with thorns and a string made of horse's hair.

6. **Defibulation:** A woman who was infibulated may be *defibulated* to allow intercourse or to give birth—this is the cutting open of her vagina once again.

> *If God wanted us to think with our wombs,*
> *why did he give us brains?*
>
> —Claire Booth Luce

—◆—

Attitudes About Female Circumcision

A 1996 report from the Egyptian Fertility Care Society, the Population Council, and Marco International showed:

1. Sixteen percent of Egyptian women are circumcised by removing the labia majora or minora, but not the clitoris. This externalizes the clitoris, much like the male glans are externalized by male circumcision.

2. Women who are circumcised are more likely to have their daughters circumcised than those who are not.

3. Women cite custom as the main reason they have their daughters circumcised.

4. Women are shifting to medical doctors to have their daughters circumcised.

5. Sixty-eight percent of women don't believe it causes complications leading to death.

6. Forty-seven percent don't believe it decreases sexual satisfaction.

7. Eighty-two percent of married and previously married women believe the practice should be continued.

I have brains and a uterus, and I use both.

—Pat Schroeder

Countries Where Female Circumcision Is Still Practiced

Australia	Indonesia
Bahrain	Kenya
Benin	Liberia
Burkina Faso	Malaysia
Cameroon	Mali
Central African Republic	Mauritania
Chad	Nigeria
Côte D'Ivoire	Senegal
Djibouti	Sierra Leone
Egypt	Somalia
Ethiopia	Sudan
Gambia	Tanzania
Ghana	Togo
Guinea	Uganda
Guinea-Bissau	United Arab Emirates
India (parts of)	Yemen

There is no doubt that the practice is a means of suppressing and controlling the sexual behavior of women. Female circumcision is a physiological chastity belt.

—Sue Armstrong

———◆———

Human Sex Hormones

Sexual behavior is influenced, sometimes quite strongly, by hormones. Here's the info on ten of the most common sex hormones.

1. **Dehydroepiandrosterone** *(DHEA)*. Manufactured by the adrenal gland, in testicles, ovaries, and brain, DHEA is the building block of other hormones. It is the most abundant hormone: In an adult man, there is about 500 times more DHEA in the bloodstream than there is testosterone. DHEA levels peak at age 25, then decline for the rest of a person's life. Supplemental DHEA (or producing more DHEA through exercise and lowering stress) may have antiaging and pro-vitality effects. DHEA produces pheromones, which can have an effect upon who you attract and are attracted to. The lower your DHEA levels, the more likely you are to be overweight. Exercising and reducing stress increase DHEA levels. Alcohol and stress lower them. You need DHEA because it increases sex drive (more in women than in men) and vitality.

2. **Dopamine.** Dopamine is a neurotransmitter (brain chemical) that increases the aggressive sex drive and makes you want sex. It allows you to feel pleasure. If you don't have dopamine, you don't feel the pleasure of anything in life. Dopamine makes you want a "high," be it sexual or otherwise. Craving for dopamine is thought to be the foundational craving of most addictions. Sexual activity increases dopamine levels. The antidepressant drug Wellbutrin also increases dopamine levels. People who like sex while they are doing it, but never think to pursue it otherwise, might be suffering from a dopamine shortage and are unable to desire the pleasure sex provides.

3. **Estrogen.** Produced by the ovaries, estrogen is in charge of the receptive sex drive in women. It makes a woman want to

say "yes" to sex. It improves bad moods and prevents depression. It promotes vaginal lubrication. A woman can increase its levels by eating soy foods and having sexual intercourse.

4. **LHRH.** Made by the hypothalamus, LHRH triggers and regulates the production of testosterone. No LHRH, no testosterone. A natural sexual stimulant, its production can be externally dependent—seeing a sexually attractive woman can trigger creation of LHRH in a man, which triggers the production of testosterone.

5. **Oxytocin.** Oxytocin is responsible for touch feeling good. It's made by the posterior pituitary gland and drives the desire to touch and be touched. It makes women want to be penetrated, increases sensitivity in the penis, and causes uterine contractions during orgasm. It promotes fast ejaculations, however. It is increased by increasing touch. It is decreased by avoiding touch and drinking alcohol.

6. **Phenylethylamine** *(PEA)*. PEA is a sexual stimulant that also works as an antidepressant. It causes romantic excitement and creates an experience of a "rush" that might make you "addicted to love." Levels increase along with romantic feelings. Chocolate contains chemicals that turn into PEA. Nutrasweet® also turns into PEA in the body and can give that "romance high."

7. **Pheromones.** Derived from DHEA, pheromones are sexual signal transmitters, and they influence whom you are sexually attracted to and who is sexually attracted to you. See the following list of "Phun Pheromone Phacts" for more on pheromones.

8. **Progesterone.** A woman's hormone—men have very little of it—progesterone is produced by the ovaries and adrenal glands. Progesterone puts the brakes on sexual desire, making a woman want sex less or not at all. It cancels out testosterone

and has been used to chemically castrate sex criminals. It's at its highest levels during the second half of the menstrual cycle.

9. **Serotonin.** Decreases sex drive. Drugs that increase serotonin (or decrease the reuptake of it in the body), such as Prozac, decrease sex drive. Along almost the same lines, it inhibits orgasm, so therefore slows down premature ejaculation. It decreases anxiousness and aggressiveness and also causes cravings for sweet foods. Women have more serotonin than men do.

10. **Testosterone.** Mostly produced by the testicles, men have 20 to 40 times more than women. Testosterone is increased by winning; so when a man feels like a loser, he is almost literally demasculinized! Testosterone motivates men's desire for separateness, while also motivating sperm production. Testosterone improves cognition, is an antidepressant, and increases sexual fantasies and desires. It increases aggressive sex drive in both men and women. Levels of testosterone surge with victory of any sort and is raised by exercise, victory, and eating meat (yes, eating meat does increase testosterone levels!). It is decreased by drinking alcohol, not exercising, and having a bad diet.

The brain is viewed as an appendage of the genial glands.

—Carl Jung

———◆———

Phun Pheromone Phacts

Pheromones are chemicals that humans and other species produce that cause a response, usually in members of the opposite sex of that species. They don't have any smell themselves, but seem to be part of the overall sexual smell of a person. If you've got the right pheromones, you can attract anyone. You are emitting them right now, along with the one thousand skin cells each centimeter of your skin slough off each hour. Here are some facts about pheromones that may interest you:

1. Some female insects produce pheromones that male insects can detect in very small quantity from very great distances. Upon detecting these pheromones the male is compelled to find the female and mate with her.

2. Women who live together, such as in a dormitory, often find that their menstrual cycles synchronize. This process appears to be governed by pheromones: Studies have shown that when a woman smells a pad that has been under another woman's arm for 24 hours, the recipient woman's menstrual cycle shifts to be closer to that of the other woman.

3. People who are aroused by the smell of a woman's or a man's worn undergarments have a sexual kink called *mysophilia*. (They also may have a higher than normal ability to detect pheromones.)

4. An English woman in Shakespeare's day would carry a "lady's apple"—a small peeled apple—in her armpit, which she would present to her man as a "love apple," full of her scent.

5. Napoleon sent a message to his love Josephine on his way home from war, telling her of his imminent arrival, and instructing her to *not* bathe. Apparently he desired her smell as much as her touch.

6. Mediterranean men dance at festivals carrying handkerchiefs in their armpits, which they wave under the noses of the women they invite to dance with them.

7. Henry III is reported to have been driven to pursue and bed a prince's wife after drying his face with a piece of her clothing and smelling her scent.

8. Research at the University of New Mexico showed that women, especially women who are ovulating, can evaluate men's level of attractiveness without seeing them—just by sniffing their worn shirts. The women would sniff the shirts and then rate the men's attractiveness; ovulating women were 50 percent more accurate than nonovulating women at correctly judging men's level of attractiveness from their smell alone.

9. A British company, Bodywise, Ltd., makes a product called Aeolus 7+, derived from pig pheromones. A mail order company in Australia used this product on collection letters they sent out—the idea being that the pheromone-saturated letters would get a stronger response from those who owed money. They sent out five hundred letters scented, and five hundred not. The scented letters were 17 percent more effective at getting people to pay.

10. Researchers do not understand human pheromones. There is no evidence that perfumes laced with pig pheromones, which are available for sale from a number of sources, have any effect on humans at all. But in the not-too-distant future, real and effective pheromone colognes may be available. Watch your nose!

I'm at the age where food has taken the place of sex in my life. In fact, I've just had a mirror put over my kitchen table.

—Rodney Dangerfield

Scents to Drive Your Partner Wild

If you can't count on having the right pheromones when you want them (and you can't, as it turns out), you might want to improve on Mother Nature through the time-tested expedient of aromatic essential oils, candles, or incense.

1. Cedar

2. Frankincense

3. Scent of ginger

4. Jasmine

5. Magnolia

6. Myrrh

7. Patchouli

8. Rose

9. Sandalwood

10. Vanilla

11. Ylang-ylang

Only the nose knows
Where the nose goes
When the door close.

—Muhammad Ali, when asked what he thought
about a boxer having sex before a big fight

———◆———

Exercises for Sexual Fitness

Exercises to develop the muscles of the pelvic floor are called "Kegal exercises." Gynecologist Arnold Kegal developed these exercises in the 1940s to help women increase the strength of the muscles around the vagina and anus—the pubococcygeal muscles, which are also known as the PC muscles.

Men and women who perform Kegal exercises have increased muscle tone in the pelvis. For women this can lead to better and stronger orgasms, for men greater control over orgasms and a feeling of sexual strength. For both men and women, these exercises can lead to increased sexual pleasure and satisfaction. Increased PC strength also helps women who "leak" urine during stressful moments.

1. Locate your PC muscles. When you go to the toilet, take a few relaxing breaths, then, while urinating with a relatively full bladder, try to stop the flow. The muscles you use to do this are your PC muscles.

2. Test your PC—muscle strength by stopping the flow of urine. How long does it take? If you can stop the flow quickly, your PC muscle is probably strong and well toned. If it takes a few seconds, or the flow only diminishes instead of stopping, you may benefit from Kegals.

3. Exercise the PC muscles using the "tense and hold" method. In this exercise you squeeze and hold your PC muscles in a contracted state, starting with three seconds and gradually working up to ten seconds. At the end of the contraction, tense the muscle "extra hard" before the release. Keep breathing during the contraction. Relax the muscles completely and breath between contractions. Work up to around 90 contractions a day.

4. Exercise the PC muscles using the rhythmic contraction method. This is also a good way to exercise and tone the PC muscles in both women and men and can help women learn to trigger orgasms. You simply contract the PC muscles over and over again, either once a second, or once every two seconds, or every three seconds. Keep breathing. At first this exercise may be difficult, but over time it will give you much greater control over your PC muscles. Repeat up to ten times, and work up to 20 sets a day.

5. Do several sets of these exercises several times daily and feel the difference.

6. Also throughout the day, tighten your stomach muscles and hold them, while breathing, for a count of five. This will help strengthen your abdominal muscles, which also are very useful during sex.

*Love is not the dying moan of a distant violin—
it's the triumphant twang of a bedspring.*

—S.J. Perelman

CHAPTER 3

Sex Industry

Sex-Industry Statistics

1. In 1992 there were 500 million adult video rentals or purchases.

2. In 1997 there were 600 million adult videos purchased or rented. That's an increase of 100 million, or of more than 270,000 a *day*.

3. *Playboy* has a circulation of 4,250,324 copies, which exceeds both *Time* and *Newsweek*.

4. In 1997 romance novels were an $855 million business.

5. In 1998 romance novels were a billion-dollar business. That's an increase of 145 million dollars, or of more than $397,000 a day!

6. Forty-five million American women read romance novels.

7. In 1998 adult Websites accounted for almost $1 billion, or 69 percent, of the worldwide revenue generated by the Internet. That number is expected to triple by 2003 and still be at least half of total Internet commerce.

8. Gay and bisexual sites account for as much as one third of the sex-related traffic on the Web.

9. There are over 8,000 adult video titles released every year. That's more than 21 a day!

The art of life lies in taking pleasures as they pass, and the keenest pleasures are not intellectual, nor are they always moral.

—Aristippus

Worldwide Statistics About Prostitutes

1. In the United States, 5,700 girls under the age of 18 are arrested annually for prostitution.

2. There are an estimated 500,000 prostitutes in Thailand, with more than over 200,000 in Bangkok alone.

3. In 1995 more than 45,000 women were arrested for prostitution in the United States.

4. More than 2 million women in the United Kingdom are, or were at some time in their lives, prostitutes.

5. On average, over 60 percent of those arrested for prostitution in the United States are white, 34 percent black, 2 percent Asian, and 1 percent Native American.

6. India has approximately 10 million prostitutes.

7. In 1996 over 60 percent of teen prostitutes arrested in the United States were male.

8. Over 70 percent of the prostitutes in Glasgow, Scotland, are drug addicts.

9. In 1997 only 96 people were arrested in the United States in rural counties for selling their bodies.

10. In France there are more than 30,000 full-time prostitutes; 95 percent of them work through pimps. There are also 60,000 part-time prostitutes.

11. In the United States, in 1997 over 47,000 people arrested for prostitution were in major urban areas. This equates to over 95 percent of the total prostitution arrests that year.

12. An estimated 70,000 Thai women have been sold to Japanese businessmen as indentured sex slaves. They are sold through brokers for around $30,000 each.

13. Prostitutes in Amsterdam, Holland, have the lowest incidence of HIV of any group of prostitutes in the world.

14. American prostitutes between the ages 23 and 39 are twice as likely to be arrested as those between the ages of 18 and 22.

15. Prostitution in Thailand generates over $4 billion per year.

16. In the United States in 1994 nearly 40 percent of all adult prostitutes arrested were male. Hence, 60 percent were female.

17. Germany has an estimated 200,000 prostitutes. Most pay income taxes, as prostitution is legally sanctioned. Nearly 65 percent of German prostitutes do so to support drug habits.

18. Around 50 percent of all Thai prostitutes are HIV positive.

Prostitution is as old as civilization. Commercial sex has survived even the most draconian and repressive attempts to eradicate it.

—Ruth Morgan Thomas, *AIDS Risks, Alcohol, Drugs and the Sex Industry* (1990)

Sex-Toy Catalogs

After reading this book you might want to purchase some sex toys to experiment with. There are hundreds of online companies that sell sex toys as well as mail order catalogs. Some of the most popu-

lar companies are listed below. If you are simply curious you may
want to contact them and get a copy of their catalog.

1. **Adam and Eve**
   (Catalog of toys, lingerie, and videos)
   P.O. Box 200
   Carrboro, NC 27510
   (800) 274-0333
   www.adameve.com

2. **Good Vibrations**
   (Highly recommended catalog of toys, books, and videos)
   1210 Valencia Street
   San Francisco, CA 94110
   (415) 974-8980
   www.goodvibes.com

3. **Eve's Garden**
   (Catalog of woman-oriented videos, toys, and books)
   119 West 57th Street, #420
   New York, NY 10019
   (212) 757-8651
   www.evesgarden.com

4. **Xandria Collection**
   (Catalog of toys, videos, and books)
   165 Valley Drive
   Brisbane, CA 94005
   (415) 468-3812
   www.xandria.com

5. **Adam's Sensual Whips and Gillian's Toys**
   (Catalog of leather and S/M resources)
   Utopian Network
   P. O. Box 1146
   New York, NY 10156
   (516) 842-1711

6. Pleasure Chest
(Catalog of toys and clothing)
7733 Santa Monica Blvd.
West Hollywood, CA 90046
(213) 650-1022

7. Drake's
(Catalog of toys and videos)
7566 Melrose Avenue
Los Angeles, CA 90046
(213) 651-5600

8. Toys in Babeland
(Catalog of videos, toys, and books)
711 East Pike Street
Seattle, WA 98122
www.babeland.com

9. Romantasy
(Catalog of lingerie, toys, books, and videos)
199 Moulton Street
San Francisco, CA 94123
(415) 673-3137

10. Holiday Products
(Catalog focused on gay audiences, includes lotions, lubricants, and novelties)
20950 Lassen Street
Chatsworth, CA 91311
(818) 772-8080

11. Blowfish Productions
(One of the best adult catalogs, featuring toys, lubes, books, and videos)
2201 Market Street, Suite 284
San Francisco, CA 94114
(800) 325-2569
www.blowfish.com

12. Erotech Corporation

(One of the largest catalogs in the United States, featuring toys, games, erotica, videos, and massage items at low prices)

1945 Carroll Avenue

San Francisco, CA 94124

(800) 748-6366

13. Male Video Direct

(Company focuses on gay videos and toys for gay men)

P.O. Box 69777

West Hollywood, CA 90069

(888) 470-7575

The best thing anyone can give a girl is a tattoo somewhere on his body with the girl's name on it. Boyfriends will come and go, but we know we'll always have each other.

—Drew Barrymore

———◆———

Where to Find a Male Escort

Finding a female prostitute is generally pretty easy. Every decent-sized town has one or several areas where prostitutes are known to hang out. In addition there are call girls, massage parlors, and other resources in which to find one. But for women to find a male escort is much more difficult. Here are several categories of male escorts that will provide the reader with a few ideas on where he or she can go tonight to look for one. The average cost for a male escort will be around $150. In some areas, they are much more expensive.

1. Male Strippers

Many male strippers are used to performing for women at bachelorette parties. They can often be hired for much more.

2. Classified Ads

Some male escorts place classified ads. In their ads they use buzz words such as "looking for wealthy women," "will travel to meet you," "discrete encounters," "seeking older women." Some male escorts place ads that simply say, "male escort available."

3. Masseuses

Some male escorts pose as massage therapists. In their ads they might mention "sensual massage" or "erotic massage." These are signs that they are likely to offer sexual services.

4. Strip Clubs for Women

Where else do male strippers hang out? They often work in strip clubs for women. Some strip clubs for men also have set nights that are just for women. Male strippers can often be hired for "private performances."

5. Swingers Clubs

Some couples enjoy hiring a man to have sex with the wife, or female partner, while the husband watches. Many men do this for free. Some swingers clubs, and other sex clubs, have male and female prostitutes available for patronage.

6. Online

Anything sexually oriented can be found online if you look hard enough. There are men online who advertise their services. Typing in the words "male escort" into a search engine will inevitably pull up loads of useless ads, but will likely also pull up some legitimate escorts who love to please.

"There's no shortage of pussy—it's just the delivery system that's messed up"

—Dr. Roy V Schenk

———◆———

12 Facts About Prostitution in Nevada

It is strange that one state in the Union has legal prostitution while everywhere else it is illegal. We have uncovered facts about the Nevada brothel scene that are strange, interesting, and will be fun facts to know at parties.

1. Nevada is the only state in America to offer legal prostitution. However, it is still illegal in Las Vegas, Reno, Carson City, and Lake Tahoe.

2. The average cost is between $150 and $500 for a session.

3. Prostitution is legal only in certain counties. Counties with large populations are forbidden from having legal prostitution.

4. It is illegal for a woman to hire a man for sex in a brothel.

5. Women who work in Nevada brothels are required to get regular medical check ups.

6. Street solicitation in Nevada is illegal. Brothels are the only place where legal prostitutes can work.

7. It is illegal for a woman to enter a brothel to obtain sex with a female prostitute.

8. There is an annual meeting of people interested in Nevada brothels. It takes place in the Carson City area. The group is called the Cyberwhoremonger Club.

9. Occasionally, famous porn stars have been known to offer their services at Nevada brothels for up to $3,000 for intercourse.

10. Nevada brothels are not allowed to advertise.

11. Those under 21 are not allowed into brothels.

12. Only a few brothels permit couples to hire a prostitute for sex. Sometimes the husband has sex with the prostitute while the wife watches. The brothel charges nearly twice as much for this option.

Prostitution sacrifices a segment of the female population in order to preserve the 'purity' of the rest.

—Abraham Kardiner, *Sex or Morality* (1955)

Worldwide Costs for a Prostitute

You asked for it, and now you've got it. Around the world the average price for a sexual experience with a prostitute greatly varies. Some countries offer prostitutes for pennies while others are very expensive. It is hard to gauge the costs, as most countries do not offer a standardization index for prostitution. As a result, we've come up with a rough index for costs. We have calculated the costs in U.S. dollars to make the guide easy to use.

1. **Australia:** Known as one of the most expensive countries in which to hire a prostitute; costs range between $150 and $600

2. **Belgium:** Between $50 and $90

3. **Canada:** Around $80 to $120 depending on city

4. **Cancun:** At least $100, but up to $800

5. **Caribbean:** Between $25 and $70

6. **China:** Approximately $30

7. **Dominican Republic:** Around $20

8. **Finland:** Around $50

9. **Germany:** Between $35 and $85

10. **Hong Kong:** Between $50 and $300, depending on age of woman

11. **Jakarta:** Between $25 and $35

12. **Japan:** Prices start around $200 and go up to $1,000+

13. **Malaysia:** Around $20

14. **Mexico:** Starting around $35

15. **Philippines:** Between $25 and $100

16. **Puerto Rico:** Between $35 and $70

17. **Russia:** Starting around $40

18. **Singapore:** Approximately $55

19. **Switzerland:** Between $20 and $60

20. **Tai Pei:** Older women charge $10 to $50, younger women charge between $50 and $200

21. **Thailand:** The average is $25 to $40

22. **Vietnam:** Between $10 and $40

Prostitutes are necessary. Without them, men would assault respectable women on the streets.

—Napolean Bonaparte

———◆———

Nevada Brothels

The ancient occupation of prostitution is alive and well in Nevada. That there are two types of brothels: the "microbrothel" and the regular brothel. The micro, as the name conveys, is smaller than the normal brothel; sometimes it's a mom-and-pop business. This list consists of some of the largest and most well-known brothels in Nevada. If you plan to visit one, it is highly recommended that you call first to make sure they are still in business and to get specific instructions on where they are located, because some are literally in the middle of nowhere. Some brothels offer limo service; others offer shuttle-bus service from large hotels. Please note that some of the (702) area code phone numbers may have been changed to (775). Also note that the average cost for a prostitute is between $100 and $500, so stock up with money before venturing out to a brothel. Good luck!

1. The Chicken Ranch
(702) 382-7870

This is one of the most famous brothels in Nevada. The ranch is named after the Broadway play *The Best Little Whorehouse in*

Texas. The Chicken Ranch is located in Pahrump, Nevada, about 50 miles from Las Vegas, off Highway 160.

2. The Mustang Ranch

The Mustang Ranch is about eight miles east of Reno on Interstate 80. It is the largest brothel in the United States. They have 30 to 50 women working at any time and have a variety of services for guests.

3. The New Sagebrush Ranch
(775) 246-5683

The New Sagebrush Ranch is located in Lyon County, approximately seven miles east of Carson City on Highway 50. They have more than 72 rooms and fantasy rooms, as well as two full-service bars. They also run an "outcall" service. The New Sagebrush is one of the most loved brothels in Nevada.

4. Mabel's Whorehouse
(702) 372-5468

Located in Crystal, in Nye County. They are in the middle of the state, off of Highway 160. This is known to be one of the nicest brothels in the area. Mabel's was built in 1985 and is designed as an Oriental-theme house. They have Japanese art on the walls and hot tubs. They also employ several Asian women.

5. The Cherry Patch II
(702) 372-5551

This well-respected brothel is located 86 miles north of Las Vegas off Highway 95 in Nye County. This is one of the closest brothels to Las Vegas. They are known for having many women under 25 working at any given time. They have a museum of prostitution and a full restaurant. They are also known for their plush rooms.

6. Moonlight Bunny Ranch

(702) 246-9901

They are located in Lyon County, approximately seven miles east of Carson City on Highway 50. They've been in business since 1956. They now have over 20 women working at any given time. They are open 24 hours a day, 365 days per year. They are known for catering to unusual sexual fantasies and kinks. Their rooms are large and plush.

7. Stardust Ranch

(702) 289-4569

They are located on High Street in Ely, White Pine County. They consider themselves a gentlemen's club and recently remodeled the entire place. The Stardust offers indoor and outdoor Jacuzzis. They also offer the option of being able to spend the night with the woman of your choice. Men love this place!

8. Salt Wells Villa

(702) 423-5335

They are located off of Highway 50, east of Fallon in Churchill County. This cathouse was opened in 1986 and is one of the only brothels in the area. This is a popular place for businessmen, cowboys, and military men. It features a Jacuzzi and an S/M playroom. It has 12 sex rooms and offers various amenities such as videos, pool table, and waterbeds. Boys as young as 14 can visit with consent from their parents. It is rumored that the women who work at Salt Wells are open to sexual experimentation.

9. Old Bridge Ranch

(702) 342-0223

They are located off of I-80, east of Reno, Exit 23. This brothel has been open since 1984 and features over 25 rooms. They have an orgy room for the wealthy and promiscuous. They also feature a collection of hundreds of porn videos for viewing pleasure. They also run an "outcall" service for those who cannot make the drive.

10. Kit Kat Ranch

(702) 246-9975

They are located in Lyon County, approximately seven miles east of Carson City on Highway 50. They customize their services for the sexual connoisseur. They offer 25 different women at any given time. They have 31 rooms, waterbeds with overhead mirrors, orgy rooms, and a spa.

The Actor and the Streetwalker . . . the two oldest professions in the world—ruined by amateurs.

—Alexander Woollcott, *Shouts and Murmurs* (1922)

The 9 Types of Prostitutes

The world of prostitution seems complicated and bizarre to those on the outside. In ancient Rome prostitutes were forced to dye their hair blond so that clients could easily identify them. At that time prostitutes were highly trained and highly paid. But now we are in much more complicated and dangerous times. In ancient Rome there were 12 types of prostitutes; from the kept woman to the beggar. Today there are nine primary categories of prostitutes.

1. Streetwalker

Streetwalkers are the most popular. Some consider this to be the lowest form of prostitution. Nearly 15 percent of women find themselves in this category. Of the streetwalkers there are four types:

a. Outlaws: those who work without a pimp

b. Rip-off artists: those who make their living from various criminal means, but prostitution is not their main form of income

c. **Thoroughbreds:** those who are new to the prostitution business and are young, attractive and act in a "professional" manner

d. **Hypes:** those who work as prostitutes to support drug habits

2. Call Girls

Call girls are of a higher caliber than streetwalkers. They tend to get paid more than streetwalkers. They generally work out of expensive hotels and tend to have regular customers. They are usually young women who are attractive and have a look of success. Around 25 percent of prostitutes fall into this category.

3. In-house Prostitutes

This type of prostitute works out of places like massage parlors, modeling agencies, brothels, or other prostitution fronts. While they are usually provided with many customers, they get paid much less than call girls, and sometimes even less than streetwalkers. Some in-house prostitutes are connected to organized crime.

4. Escort-Service Prostitutes

There has been a new wave of prostitutes who advertise in the Yellow Pages and in newspapers, magazines, and so forth as escort services. These companies have many women who travel to hotels, homes, or anywhere else to provide men with "sensual massage," companionship, or other sexually oriented activity. Since the women work for a company they tend to be paid less than call girls, but make more money than both in-house prostitutes and streetwalkers because they tend to have sex with wealthy men.

5. Drug Addicted and Homeless Prostitutes

These prostitutes depend on clients to support their drug habits. As a result they tend to deal with men who are more likely to abuse and harm them. They are more likely to acquire AIDS, for example, and are much more likely to be beaten up or hurt.

It is estimated that 50 percent of teen prostitutes are drug addicts.

Homeless prostitutes find themselves in a similar desperate situation as do drug addicts. They are often runaways who have nowhere to go. As a result they become prostitutes to survive. They run a high risk of being beaten up, raped, arrested or exposured to STDs and HIV.

6. Part-time Prostitutes

Some women, including mothers, students, and housewives, turn to prostitution to make extra money. These women use prostitution as a way to make quick money when they need it. The numbers of part-timers are increasing.

7. Professional Dominatrixes

Many professional dominatrixes engage in the basic bondage and discipline activities: sadism, masochism, bondage, whips, chains, and erotic power exchange between themselves and submissive men. A real dominatrix is involved in sadism and masochism and psychological torture, but does not include genital touching in the process. Other women, however, use domination as a prostitution front. Many women who call themselves dominatrixes are in fact obtaining clients under a more legally protected title and, in fact, engage in sexual intercourse and other sexual interactions. Dominatrixes tend to be paid nearly as much as call girls. The average domination session costs $125 to $500 per hour.

8. Indentured Sex Slaves

Indentured sex slaves are girls and women who are forced into prostitution to repay debts, or sometimes just because they are threatened. This type of prostitution is fairly common in Third World countries, but there have also been several cases in the United States.

9. Madams

Madams manage other women. They tend to run brothels or escort services. Some also work part-time as prostitutes, but in general they work with clients and sell their prostitutes. Many madams tend to be over 40 and former call girls.

It is a silly question to ask a prostitute why she does it . . . These are the highest paid "professional" women in America.

—Gail Sheehy, *Hustling* (1971)

———◆———

Addresses of 30 Porn Stars

Everyone loves a porn star. The modern starlets are used to receiving tons of mail from horny men. If you are interested in contacting stars you've seen, read about, or obsessed about, here they are in alphabetical order:

1. **Ginger Lynn Allen,** 6520 Platt Avenue #811, West Hills, CA 91307

2. **Danni Ashe,** 520 Washington Blvd, #445, Marina del Rey, CA 90292. E-mail: www.danni.com

3. **Juli Ashton,** 9800 D Topanga Canyon Blvd., #352, Chatsworth, CA 91311. E-mail: juliashton@risque.com

4. **Christy Canyon,** 13601 Ventura Blvd., #218, Sherman Oaks, CA 91423

5. **Marilyn Chambers,** 4526 W. Charleston Blvd. #836, Las Vegas, NV 89102

6. **Annabel Chong,** C/O D.O.M. Corporation, P.O. Box 9786, Marina del Rey, CA 90295

7. **Raquel Darrian,** 9101 W. Sahara Ave. Suite 105-B12, Las Vegas, NV 89117

8. **Vanessa Del Rio,** 309 Fifth Ave, Suite 234, Brooklyn, NY 11215

9. **Nina Hartley,** 1442A Walnut, #242, Berkeley, CA 94709

10. **Houston,** Alley Katz Enterprises, 9899 Santa Monica Blvd., Suite 606, Beverly Hills, CA 90212

11. **Kylie Ireland,** 9800D Topanga Canyon Blvd, #352, Chatsworth, CA 91311

12. **Jenna Jameson,** 9800D Topanga Canyon Blvd., #343, Chatsworth, CA 91311

13. **Jill Kelly,** 207 West Los Angeles Ave, Suite 134, Moorpark, CA 93021

14. **Chasey Lain,** 9800D Topanga Canyon Blvd., #352, Chatsworth, CA 91311

15. **Christi Lake,** 19528 Ventura Blvd, #565, Tarzana, CA 91356

16. **Hypatia Lee,** 15127 Califa St., Van Nuys, CA 91401

17. **Amber Lynn,** 12400 Ventura Blvd. #329, Studio City, CA 91604-2406

18. **Porsche Lynn,** 12439 Magnolia Blvd., #203, N. Hollywood, CA 91607

19. **Madison,** C/O 4 Ugly Women, P.O. Box 8424-A, Santa Monica Blvd, Suite 173, West Hollywood, CA 90069

20. **Anna Malle,** P.O. Box 97833, Las Vegas, NV 89193. E-mail: annamalle@annamalle.com

21. **Midori,** 7095 Hollywood Blvd, #823, Hollywood, CA 90028. www.XXXMidori.com/ E-mail: xxxmidori@aol.com

22. **Chessie Moore,** P.O. Box 577, Satsuma, FL 32189-0577. Email: cmoore@funport.net

23. **Tiffany Mynx,** 1534 N. Moorpark Rd, #309, Thousand Oaks, CA 91360

24. **Roni Raye,** P. O. Box 11717, Indianapolis, IN 46201. E-mail: roniraye@roniraye.com, www.roniraye.com

25. **Alicia Rio,** 1840 S. Gaffey St., #165, San Pedro, CA 90730

26. **Rocki Roads,** P. O. Box 285163, Boston, MA 02128-5163

27. **Savannah Memorial Fan Club,** 11225 Magnolia Blvd, Penthouse, N. Hollywood, CA 91601

28. **Seka,** 5-K Sales, 1122 White Rock, Dixon, IL 61021

29. **Marilyn Star,** 1521 Alton Rd, #369, Miami Beach, FL 33139

30. **Ona Zee,** 4724 Lincoln Blvd, #320, Marina del Rey, CA 90292

My reaction to porno films is as follows: After the first ten minutes I want to go home and screw. After the first twenty minutes, I never want to screw again as long as I live.

—Erica Jong

Phone Sex 101: Facts, Rumors, and Information

The past 15 years has seen the emergence of phone sex. In that time phone sex has become an extremely popular sexual outlet.

Open up most magazines and you will find advertisement after advertisement for phone sex services. Phone sex is a popular subject among comedians. Even the cartoon figures Beavis and Butthead once called a phone sex line. We've compiled several facts, rumors, and other information about this new industry.

1. On her famous *20/20* appearance with Barbara Walters, Monica Lewinsky mentioned that she and Clinton enjoyed phone sex together.

2. In 1999 between $4 and $5 billion was spent on phone sex.

3. In Corpus Christi, Texas, the U.S. Department of Housing and Urban Development distributed a flyer to 46,000 residents on how citizens could obtain free public housing. However, they made a mistake and placed the wrong toll-free phone number—it was a phone-sex line. Whoops!

4. On average, 50 percent of people who call 900 numbers avoid paying for them.

5. In April 2000 a judge in Munich, Germany, convicted a former German state legislator of defrauding taxpayers. Hans Wallner, 48, was found guilty of making over 405 phone sex calls and running up over $15,000 in debt. He was ordered to pay $11,000 to a German charity and was suspended from his job for 15 months.

6. The average phone-sex operator is paid $12 per hour.

7. Phone sex became legal in 1982 after telephone deregulation.

8. In 1997 a 25-year-old man was arrested for stealing from his boss. The man stole $37,000 to pay his phone bill. The man had been spending over 90 minutes per day, every day, calling telephone sex numbers and was terribly in debt.

9. Experts estimate that over 500,000 phone sex calls are made in the United States each day.

10. In 1999 the telecommunications minister of Saudi Arabia blocked access in all political offices from using sex lines. The phone sex block was done after a single customer had charged up a phone bill of $345,000 in phone sex calls. The minister found another customer who had several phone bills over $80,000. Within six months of beginning their antiphone sex campaign they had blocked access to more than 50 phone sex lines.

11. The average phone sex call costs between $1.99 and $4.99 per minute. The average call costs between $25 and $100.

12. One Greenwich, Connecticut phone-company employee could not wait to get home to participate in phone sex, so he found a way to call 900-number phone sex lines while at work. He also found a way to charge the costs to Bell-Atlantic customers in New York, Connecticut, and New Jersey. He charged up over $70,000.

13. According to phone sex operator Roni Raye, there are several common sex fantasies when calling a phone sex line. Men of all professions call phone lines; Raye claims to have had several politicians, including a senator, call her line. Surprisingly, Raye says that many men call because they are lonely, and they just want to talk to someone, often not about sexual topics.

    Here are the top ten fantasies for men calling phone sex line:

    • Oral sex

    • The man being anally penetrated by a woman

    • The man submitting to the woman

    • Domination and humiliation

- Straight sex

- The man giving oral sex

- The man having sex with more than one woman at a time

- The man being watched as he has sex with the phone sex operator

- The man having sex with a much younger woman

- Spanking, beating, or other sadistic desires

There is some good news and some bad news. The bad news is that state employees from 84 agencies racked up more than a thousand dollars in telephone calls to pornographic recordings in New York. The good news is that none came from the Governor's mansion.

—Press secretary to former Virginia governor Charles Robb, upon discovering a noticeable increase in state phone bills during 1983

———◆———

Magazines About the Adult Movie Industry

1. AVN

9414 Eton Street, Chatsworth, CA 91311 (818) 718-5788. E-mail: www.avn.com

This magazine is clearly the best magazine on the topic available. They have hundreds of reviews in each issue. They focus on many types of adult films including gay, bondage, amateur, and professional. They also include interesting legal information and news about the pornography industry.

2. Hustler Erotic Video Guide

P.O. Box 16507, North Hollywood, CA 91615

This magazine is published by Larry Flynt Publications. The magazine is mostly ads and pictures of adult stars. There is very little editorial content. The subscription rate is $39.95 for 12 issues.

3. Batteries Not Included

C/O Richard Freeman, 130 Limestone Street, Yellow Springs, OH 45387. E-mail: bni@aol.com

Freeman is a freelancer who writes adult video reviews for several porn magazines, so we know he is well versed in the ways of the adult video. This magazine contains interviews with many adult stars as well as a solid number of video reviews. The cost is $3 per issue, and he publishes 12 issues per year.

4. Homefront

4230 East Towne Blvd., Suite 287, Madison, WI 53704

Homefront magazine is all about the amateur porn industry. It is crude and rude and makes no apologies about its antigloss, no-holds-barred approach. They include several interviews with amateur stars and dozens of video reviews with each issue. The cost is $7.50 for a sample issue.

5. Screw

Milky Way Productions, Inc., P.O. Box 432, Old Chelsea Station, New York, NY 10011

This magazine is published by the infamous Al Goldstein. The magazine comes out weekly and is mostly available in porn stores across the United States. This tabloid-style newspaper features a minimal amount of articles or content and is filled with phone sex ads and other tripe that generate revenue for Goldstein.

They are known to push the First Amendment laws and to feature controversial articles to push limits. They do feature adult video reviews and dedicate a fair amount of space to discussing adult videos.

6. Adam Film World
8060 Melrose Avenue, Los Angeles, CA 90046

This magazine has been in publication since the late 1960s. They publish 12 issues per year and do a good job of covering the adult world. They review many films in each issue, feature stills, and often have trading cards and large posters in the magazine. Each year they also publish the *Annual Directory of Adult Films,* which is arguably the best source available.

Subscriptions cost $45, and the *Annual Directory* costs $10.50.

7. Video Xcitement
P.O. Box 187, Frasier, MI 48026

This newspaper focuses on amateur films. They produce a nonglossy, amateur-looking magazine that is thorough and features a large amount of editorial content. Subscriptions cost $36 for 12 issues.

8. Adult Stars Magazine
1008 West Hallandale Beach Blvd, Hallandale, FL 33009. (954) 458-0021

This magazine offers many photos and interviews with adult stars from the 1970s to today. They are known for having interesting articles and good film reviews.

> *. . . pornographic magazines are the fifth most frequently discarded item in hotels.*
>
> —Guardian (November 25, 1992)

———◆———

Prostitute Support Groups

1. Coyote

2269 Chestnut St. #452, San Francisco, CA 94123

The leading organization in the United States for prostitution support and legal reform issues.

2. Prostitutes of New York

25 West 45th Street, #1401, New York, NY 10036

They offer counseling and suggestions on how to get out of the business.

3. Hooking Is Real Employment

P.O. Box 98386, Atlanta, GA 39359

Another national lobbying group for the legalization of prostitution and for prostitution rights.

4. Prostitutes Anonymous

11225 Magnolia Blvd., #181, North Hollywood, CA 91601

This group helps women get out of prostitution and offers support and counseling.

*Prostitution is hard, if not impossible,
to eradicate. Everywhere men (and women)
seek sexual gratification and are willing
to pay for it. Accordingly, every society
has to compromise, to find a way to contain
this "necessary evil."*

—P.U. Venema, *Safer Prostitution: A New
Approach in Holland*

———◆———

Nevada "Microbrothels"

There are many small "mom-and-pop" brothels in Nevada that are locally run and owned. Just as microbreweries often have the best beer, many of the smaller brothels have the best women and most interesting atmosphere. This list consists of the smaller brothels, which are said to be more interesting than the larger ones, but also more inconsistent. They certainly have personality.

1. Sharon's Place
(702) 754-6427

They are located off State Route 278, I-80 exit in Elko County. This microbrothel is custom-made for truckers. They feature free coffee and showers. The parking lot is designed to handle semi-trucks. Sharon's is open 24 hours per day.

2. Billie's Ranch

This microbrothel is located in Tonopah, in Mineral County, South of Mina, off Highway 95. They are near the Test Range Military Site, 207 miles northwest of Las Vegas. Billie's is literally a trailer in the middle of nowhere, with a bartender and two working girls. They have been in business since 1975. They do not have a phone, but are said to be open 24 hours per day.

3. Donna's
(775)-752-9959; E-mail: www.donnasranch.com

They are located in Wells, off Highway 80. This small brothel was owned by prizefighter Jack Dempsey in the 1940s. They have been in business for 160 years. They cater to truckers and have between two and four women working at any given time.

4. Mona Lisa
(702) 738-9923

They are located in Elko in Elko County, off Highway 95, on Douglas Street. This brothel has been in business for over 70 years.

They have a small operation, but are known to feature very attractive women and X-rated films.

5. Bobbies Buckeye Bar

(702) 482-9984

Tonopah, Nye County. Bobbies is located off Highway 6 a few miles east of Tonopah. The sign behind the bar reads, "pussy is better than hamburger," so you know that these guys are serious about the brothel business. They are located in the same spot as the first Nevada brothel. Bobbies has a relaxed environment. They are one of the last places in Nevada not to accept credit cards.

6. My Place

(702) 623-9919

They are located in Winnemucca, in Humbolt County. Several brothels are located on Baud Street in Winnemucca (My Place, Simones De Paris, Villa Joy, and Penny's Cozy Corner). My Place is supposedly one of the friendliest cathouses in Nevada. It is run by Madam Barbara Davis, who was once given the prestigious award of "Number One Madam in Nevada."

7. Kitty's Guest Ranch

(702) 246-9810

They are located in Lyon County, approximately seven miles east of Carson City on Highway 50. Kitty Bono (no relation to Sonny) is the owner and full-time madam at Kitty's. She designed the ranch and has been running it since 1979. She usually has six women working at a time. Kitty has been in the business for over 30 years. She once worked as a madam for Joe Conforte. Conforte was known for his portable brothels, which would be moved across county lines to avoid police problems. Kitty's offers "outcall" services and is open 24 hours per day.

8. Lazy B Guest Ranch

(702) 423-3221

They are located east of Fallon, off Highway 50 in Churchill County. This just might be the smallest microbrothel of them all.

They usually have two women working at any given time. The atmosphere is relaxed, and they have a bar with video machines and pool tables. They rely on Navy personnel as their prime customer base; Fallon is on a bombing run. Lazy B also allows service to 16-year-olds, but no alcohol.

9. The Pussycat
(702) 623-9939

The Pussycat is one of four brothels located in Winnemucca, in Humbolt County. This brothel, however, is the oldest of them all. They opened in the 1800s. The bar is decorated in the familiar Western theme with wooden floors and a saloon atmosphere. They feature between five and ten women at any given time. They are open 24 hours per day.

> *I believe that sex is the most beautiful, natural, and wholesome thing that money can buy.*
>
> —Steve Martin

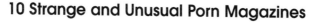

10 Strange and Unusual Porn Magazines

This list includes magazines that are homemade and printed in very limited quantities. They tend to be about fetishes and uncommon topics.

1. Eidos: Sexual Freedom and Erotic Entertainment for Women and Men
P.O. Box 96
Boston, MA 02137
E-mail: eidos@eidos.org
www.eidos.org

Eidos is known for its ability to push sexual limits and provide taboo article after taboo article. *Eidos* focuses on extreme S/M, as well as First Amendment sex issues. Editor Brenda Lowe has been publishing this magazine for over six years and it continues to expand and improve. She offers many book, sex magazine, and video reviews as well. Subscription rates are $45 for 8 issues or $5 for a sample issue.

2. Underliners

Sasha's Studio
P.O. Box 12398
Seattle, WA 98111

No matter what your kink or fetish, there is probably a magazine or a fan club that already exists for those who share the same desires. *Underliners* is a journal that focuses solely on bras and is dedicated to bra enthusiasts everywhere. Some issues discuss the types of bras, other issues the history of bras. Stories, letters, and current trends in the industry are also included. There are even pictures of bras. The cost for a subscription is $15 for 6 issues.

3. WhaP: Women Who Administer Punishment

Retro Systems
P.O. Box 69491
Los Angeles, CA 90069
E-mail: whap@hooked.net

WhaP is one of the most engaging and fun to read magazines about S/M available. They focus on providing information to women on how to dominate and train their husbands and boyfriends. However, they do so in a fun and often humorous manner. Each issue features celebrity advice on training men as well as photos from 1940s and 1950s fetish magazines. The cost for a subscription is $29 for four issues.

4. Smoke Signals: A Monthly Journal Devoted to the Smoking Fetish

500 Waterman Avenue, Suite 193

E. Providence, RI 02914

E-mail: SmokeSigs@aol.com

www.smokesigs.com

Does it turn you on to watch women smoke? Well, some men have a smoking fetish and this journal caters to their needs. As you can guess, there are very few magazines that focus on smoking, so this type of journal is a rarity. Stories, letters, and photos are included in this 20-page monthly newsletter. The subscription cost is $49.95 for 12 issues.

5. Celebrate the Self: The Magazine of Solo Sex

C/O Robert Bahr

Factor Press

P.O. Box 8888

Mobile, AL 36689

Do you enjoy masturbating? If so, then this may be the magazine for you. The magazine is aimed at men who want to learn new and exciting breakthrough techniques in the ancient art of self-pleasure. While the magazine has a gay slant, men of all sexual preferences can find something interesting and even useful. Subscriptions cost $24.95 for six issues.

6. DeSade Magazine

C/O Vanilla Christ

P.O. Box 1394

Burlington, VT 05402

DeSade magazine focuses on S/M practices and does a good job with solid editorial content. They also provide hot and sexy fetish photos and interviews with female dominants and submissives. One of the best parts of the magazine is that they occa-

145

sionally list shops and catalogs around the world that sell fetish toys.

7. Hair to Stay: The Magazine for Lovers of Natural, Hairy Women

Pam Winter

P.O. Box 80667

South Dartmouth, MA 02748

E-mail: pam@hairtostay.com

The premise of this magazine is that women have the right to be as hairy as they want. This means facial, armpit, leg, and even ass hair. The other purpose this magazine serves is to provide men who fantasize about hairy women an opportunity for pictures and stories about such women. This magazine is professionally made and is well respected. Subscriptions run $40 for four issues.

8. Fascination

Bette Hagglund

3949 W. Irving Park Road

Chicago, IL 60618

This magazine is one of the more unusual of the bunch—it is about amputee fantasies and desires. It contains many fictional tales of sex with amputees as well as photos of amputee women. Occasionally there are first-person accounts of sex from an amputee's point of view. Subscriptions cost $50 for four issues.

9. Loving More: New Models for Relationships

P.E.P. Publishing

P.O. Box 4358

Boulder, CO 80306

E-mail: ryam@lovemore.com

www.lovemore.com

This magazine provides for people interested in polyamory; that is, having intimate relations with more than one person at a time. *Loving More* offers advice to people on how they can maintain more than one loving relationship at a time. They offer space for classified and personals ads and other network opportunities. The magazine preaches many New-Age philosophies of love and harmony within relationships. Subscriptions run $24 for four issues.

10. HE-SHE
Continental Spectator
P.O. Box 278
Canal Street Station
New York, NY 10013

What list of fetishes would be complete without the inclusion of male sissy babies and submissive transsexuals and transvestites? *HE-SHE* offers photos, articles, and stories about submissive men. Occasionally they run articles on how to become a transvestite or a drag queen. Each issue includes personal ads and phone sex ads for men who love transsexuals and transvestites. The cost is $10 per issue.

> *If the sex scene doesn't make you want to do it — whatever it is they're doing — it hasn't been written right.*
>
> —Sloan Wilson

———◆———

Conventions for Swingers

There are several conventions and weekend-long events designed for people interested in swinging to come together and experience the fun and raw sexual fury of the ever-popular swinging.

1. The Annual Lifestyles Convention

For information, contact: Lifestyles Organization, 2641 LaPalma Avenue, Suite B, Anaheim, CA 92801 (714) 821-9953, www.PlayCouples.com

This convention is the largest and oldest of its kind. In 1996 over 3,000 people attended. HBO covered the event for their "Real Sex" show. The Lifestyles Convention offers seminars and workshops on swinging as well as a large marketplace exhibition hall.

2. The Visions Convention

Contact: Holly and Ray, P.O. Box 12457, Ft. Pierce, FL 34979 (561) 460-6649

This convention is sponsored by the publishers of the swingers magazine *Contact Socials*. This convention is relatively small, but offers seminars on erotic topics and time to socialize. The convention takes place in Florida as an opportunity for a winter vacation. They usually book an entire hotel. The Visions Convention is known for its party atmosphere and fun times.

3. Friendship Express Travel

Contact: Toni and Glen, Friendship Express, P.O. Box 581515, Minneapolis, MN 55458. E-mail: toni.and.glen@tfexp. xom, http://tfexp.com

Glen and Toni run a swingers club called Club H. They sponsor several weekend getaway trips, parties, and trips for those involved in swinging. Their schedule is constantly being updated, so contact them directly for the schedule of upcoming events.

4. The Annual Conclave Convention

Contact: Mike Conclave, P.O. Box 110, Mt. Zion, IL 60056, (847) 297-4711. E-mail: exnocon@ix.netcom.com, www.lifestyle. com/execswing

This convention has been running yearly for nearly 20 years. Couples and single women come together at this event sponsored by the North Swing Club in Chicago. Around 300 to 450 couples attend each spring. As usual there are seminars, and each night there are dances. They usually offer a suite for those interested in bondage, S/M, and other kinky delights.

5. Hedonism

http://www.supernclubs.com/hedonism.html

Hedonism is an annual event that takes place in Jamaica. This famous convention offers nude events, live sex on stage, bathing-suit contests, and much more. Many groups of kinky folks from around the world gather at this event. There are many swingers that attend as well as nudists.

6. Elite International's Ball

Contact: Elite International, P.O. Box 22728, Nashville, TN 37202, (615) 244-2438

These semi-annual balls usually have between 100 and 150 couples in attendance. They are designed to be relaxed and informal gatherings of couples interested in meeting other couples for the purpose of swinging.

I believe that sex is a beautiful thing between two people. Between five, it's fantastic.

—Woody Allen

---◆---

Sex Jobs

1. Sex Surrogate

Sex surrogates are neither prostitutes nor gigolos. They work as sex educators, teachers, therapists, and lovers. While they do on occasion have sexual intercourse with their patients, the act is done within a therapeutic context. Sex surrogates mainly work with men and women who have sexual problems.

2. Female Deflowerer

In parts of South America virgins are not allowed to be married. The government hires men to travel from village to village to assist women in losing their virginity so that they can then become married.

3. Sushi Geisha

In parts of Japan attractive young women are hired for a traditional feast called *nyotaimoro,* sometimes translated as "the adorned body of a woman." Wealthy businessmen eat sushi off naked virgins. The cost is usually $1,200 per virgin. The meals can last up to eight hours. The women must remain perfectly still and are trained by having eggs and ice cubes placed on their bodies to build up their endurance.

4. Sexual Mommy

Many men enjoy pretending they are adult babies. They wear diapers, drink milk from a bottle, and are often breast fed by "sexual mommies." These women do not have sexual intercourse with the babies. Sexual mommies do not even usually touch the genitalia of adult babies. Some women who work as professional dominatrixes perform these types of scenes as well.

5. Fluffer

A fluffer is someone who works on pornographic movie sets and is hired to ensure that the male stars have an erect penis when they go onto the set for filming. Fluffers often perform oral sex on male stars and occasionally they have intercourse with them as well.

6. Dating Coach

A dating coach is someone skilled in the art of seduction. They work with men and women on how to develop skills in this area. For example, the authors of this book, David Copeland and Ron Louis, run a dating institute where they work with men and women and help them create their dream relationships. The work is usually done through experiential exercises, conversation, homework, and through other emotionally oriented work. To find out more about their coaching and/or workshops check them out on the web:

www.howtosucceedwithwomen.com (*for men*), and
www.howtosucceedwithmen.com (*for women*).

You can also write to them: P.O. Box 55094, Madison, WI 53705 or at succeed@pobox.com

7. Dominatrix

To be a dominatrix a woman has to be versed in many different styles of domination, from forced feminization to light bondage, from training a man to be a dog through dealing with religious issues around sexual liberation. Some dominatrixes also have sex with their clients. Others command the men to masturbate. A dominatrix deals with a large variety of sexual desires, fantasies, and fetishes.

8. Genitalia Instructor

In nearly every medical school people are hired to train medical students in how to give gynecological exams, prostate exams, and hernia exams. While this certainly is not overtly sexual, obviously it involves the sex organs. Female instructors teach students exactly how to open the vaginal lips and how deep to insert fingers when checking for potential problems. Male instructors show and tell students how far to insert fingers into the anus to check the prostate.

9. Toilet Model

We interviewed one woman who made her living making videos of herself going to the bathroom. No masturbation or any overt sexual contact, just sitting on the toilet going to the bathroom. She made over $50,000 per year selling the videos.

*Sexual intercourse is kicking death
in the ass while singing.*

—Charles Bukowski

———◆———

CHAPTER 4

Law

Censorships Around the World

1. Argentina

Argentina is a highly Catholic country. However, they have very little censorship. Pornography is widely available. Films are classified by age, but are not censored. Television has soft porn on cable channels. Music is not censored, nor are theatres.

2. Belgium

Belgium is one of the most progressive countries in Europe. They have no censorship laws at all. There is no legal definition of pornography. However, the government can seize materials that outrage public decency. The government rarely makes arrests for pornography. Pornography is on television after 10:00 P.M. State and local television stations ban ads for drugs and contraceptives, however. Magazines and newspapers are not censored.

3. Canada

Canadian censorship laws are similar to those in the United States, but stricter. Pornography is available in sex shops. However, the State-run Customs Department seizes much of the porn that is sent to Canada. Pornography is not allowed on cable TV; both television and radio are highly censored. Several years ago there was a lawsuit against several stores for selling *Playboy* magazine. The suit claimed that the magazine created a hostile environment for female customers. Rock music is not censored, though parental-warning stickers are required.

4. Egypt

Egypt is known as the most liberal Muslim nation. However, censorship has been strictly enforced since the Egyptian revolution in 1955. Since then, Egypt has been controlled by the military. Production and distribution of pornography is illegal. Many Egyptians have access to porn through satellites, and, as a result, the government is considering outlawing satellite dishes. Many foreign films are cut or banned when they reach Egypt. Sex scenes are frequently removed from films. On television all scenes involving kissing or other sexual activities are removed. Foreign books and magazines are often banned, and rock music that has sexual overtones and lyrics can be banned. For example, Madonna and George Michael are banned from all Egyptian radio stations.

5. France

France's censorship laws tend to be minimal. Only violent pornography is banned. Hardcore pornography videos are sold in adult shops and regular supermarkets. Pornography is on cable TV. Anything can be advertised on TV; films are not censored; art galleries are uncensored. Newspapers and magazine are also uncensored.

6. Germany

The constitution in Germany prohibits censorship. Some movies are banned because they glorify violence. Certain books are banned because they promote fascism or racism. Hardcore pornography is banned and so are bondage pictures or photos of erect penises. Sex is available on television, but not hardcore sex. Many films are banned for either sexual or violent content. Most films are edited before they are shown on television. Over 700 books are banned, most violent or drug related. Many punk-rock groups are banned from selling their music in Germany. Prostitution is legal in parts of Germany, however.

7. Iceland

Iceland can be quite conservative in its views toward public censorship. However, there are very few prosecutions in censorship cases. Pornography is not sold, but can be picked up by satellite. Swedish and Danish pornography magazines are sold in Iceland. Many films are banned or edited if they have strong sexual content. Newspapers and magazines are uncensored.

8. India

India houses the largest movie industry in the world. However, no kissing or other sexual activity is allowed on the screen. Furthermore, vulgarity is also prohibited. Pornography is illegal and unavailable. Television is self-censored. Newspapers as well as magazines are generally not censored. Some theaters have had performances stopped as a result of public outrage, but they are not formally censored.

9. Ireland

The strict religious code of Ireland has spilled over into the area of censorship. Ireland is restricted by several censorship codes. Pornography is illegal in every medium. However, there are sex shops in Dublin that sell soft-core pornography. Many movies are banned or edited because of sex or violence. The radio is censored from discussing overtly sexual topics. Newspapers are heavily censored by the government. Several art galleries have been fined for sexual art.

10. Israel

Israel continues to function with very little censorship. Pornography is available on cable television as well as in sex shops across the country. Furthermore, there are no restrictions about which products can or cannot be advertised on television. No program has been censored on Israeli television since the 1970s. The only book that has been, and remains, banned is *Mein Kampf* by Adolf Hitler. Films are rarely censored, nor is music. Art is not censored. In fact controversial art is embraced. One of the largest exhibits ever of Robert Mapplethorpe was in Tel Aviv.

11. Japan

While Japan is very lenient with how they monitor violence in the media, they are much more strict with laws pertaining to sexuality. Even cultural norms are quite conservative. For example, couples rarely kiss or even hold hands in public. Sex in the arts is censored. Frontal nudity in magazines is against the law. Pornography is illegal, except for Japanese bondage movies. Books are censored, as are newspapers. Radio stations are also censored. On the other hand, there are no laws against cruelty toward animals.

12. United Kingdom

England has fairly strict censorship laws. Artists, writers, and video collectors are the most likely to be censored and affected. Public art galleries have frequently been shunned by officials. Pornography remains illegal, but much is sold on the black market. Videos are routinely banned for sexual scenes. Many television shows are also banned and edited because of sex. Music is rarely banned. However, music videos are banned and censored for sexual content.

> *Censorship reflects society's lack of confidence in itself.*
>
> —Potter Stewart

Worldwide Prostitution Guide: Countries Where Prostitution Is Legal and Illegal

Throughout the world there are brothels and other places of prostitution. In some places, such as Amsterdam, there are infamous red-light districts. In many countries where prostitution is legal, health checkups are required. If you are considering hiring a prostitute, you should be aware that there is a worldwide health crisis among prostitutes; many are infected with HIV. In countries such as India, approximately 30 percent of prostitutes have HIV. Countries in Southern Asia have a much higher incidence of HIV. A good rule of thumb when dealing with prostitutes is that if they do not require you to wear a condom, then you should not have sex with them.

Countries Where Prostitution Is Legal

Argentina	Indonesia
Aruba	Italy
Australia	Mexico
Belgium	Norway
Belize	Parts of England
Cancun	Peru
Chile	Philippines
Cuba	Portugal
Ecuador	Scotland
Germany	Singapore
Greece	Sweden
Guam	Switzerland
Holland	Venezuela

Countries Where Prostitution Is Accepted, But Not Regulated

Cambodia	France
Canada	Honduras
China	Hong Kong
Costa Rica	Japan
Czechoslovakia	Korea
Denmark	Nicaragua
Finland	Panama

Poland

Puerto Rico

Russia

Santa Domingo

Spain

Taiwan

Thailand

Countries Where Prostitution Is Illegal

Bahaman Islands

Bermuda

Jamaica

United States (except Nevada)

Vietnam

Virgin Islands

Yugoslavia

Ignorant laws, ignorant prejudices, ignorant codes or morals, condemn one portion of the female sex to vicious excess, another to as vicious restraint, and generally the whole of the male sex to debasing licentiousness, if not loathsome brutality.

—Frances Wright (1827)

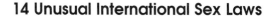

14 Unusual International Sex Laws

1. In Tasmania widows are required to wear their dead husband's penis around their neck for a period of time after his death. A similar law is enforced in Gippsland, Australia.

2. An ancient law in Indonesia prohibited men from masturbating. The punishment was decapitation.

3. In Wrokaw, Poland, wives are allowed to beat or kill any woman who is sleeping with their husband. She can either beat the woman to death or just wound her unmercifully. However, the only weapon she may use is a club.

4. In Bhutan a younger brother is not allowed to lose his virginity before his older brother. Furthermore, a younger brother may not marry before his older brother.

5. In Peru men are not allowed to have sex with female alpaca.

6. In Uruguay, men cannot touch their wives during their menstrual period. If convicted of this crime, a man can be fined and publicly whipped 200 times or more.

7. In Iran married men can legally have homosexual sex with their wife's father, brother, or son.

8. If a husband catches his wife in bed with another man in Uruguay, he is given several options on how to handle the situation under the law. One option is to kill the wife and her lover. No further questions asked. The other option is to castrate the man with a knife and then slice off the nose from his wife. Which option would you choose?

9. In Yemen, prostitution is illegal. Women convicted are publicly beheaded.

10. Rapists in Nambia have choices. If convicted of rape a man can either choose castration or 20 years of hard labor.

11. Several Middle Eastern Islamic countries have laws stating that it is illegal to eat meat from a sheep you have had sex with.

12. In Suriname a widow must first have sex with a member of her deceased husband's family before she can remarry.

13. Men were taxed as a punishment for having sex with animals in Ancient Rome.

14. In Communist China, anyone caught distributing pornography is sentenced to death.

The goal of sexual repression is to produce an individual who is adjusted to the authoritarian order and will submit to it in spite of all misery and degradation.

—William Reich, *The Mass Psychology of Fascism*

———◆———

Divorce: Words, Laws, and Facts

- "You never really know a man until you have divorced him."
  —Zsa Zsa Gabor

- In Smelterville, Idaho, a man divorced his wife because she dressed up as a ghost and tried to scare his mother out of their house. The man won the divorce.

- Over 50 percent of marriages result in divorce.

- A Hawaii man filed for divorce because his wife was a pea freak. She served him pea soup for breakfast and made pea sandwiches for his lunch.

- "Always get married early in the morning. That way if it doesn't work out, you haven't wasted the whole day."
  —Mickey Rooney

- In Roman times women often divorced men simply because they were bored.

- According to the Janus Report, couples who lived together before marriage are more likely to get divorced after marriage.

- A Chicago woman filed for divorce after her husband refused to turn off the TV during a football game and make love.

- "There are four stages to a marriage. First there's the affair, then marriage, then children, and finally the fourth stage, without which you cannot know a woman, the divorce.
  —Norman Mailer

- Among divorced couples most men divorced women because of sexual reasons. Most women divorced men because of an extra-marital affair.

- A New Mexico woman divorced her husband because he forced her to call him "Major" and then salute him each time she walked by.

  "The night before, Burt told me I was the love of his life . . . The next morning I was served with divorce papers."
  —Loni Anderson

- The early Catholic Church banned divorced. They allowed people to separate, but to never remarry.

- Thomas Mihalck, 38, and Ann Mello, 34, had a brief marriage. During their wedding party Mihalck became furious when Mello danced with a man at the party. He started beating Mello and was later arrested. She filed for divorce the next day.

I am a marvelous housekeeper. Every time I leave a man, I keep his house.

—Zsa Zsa Gabor

Laws That Regulate Oral and Anal Sex

1. **Alabama:** Oral or anal sex with someone other than one's spouse is illegal and punishable by a one-year jail term.

2. **Arizona:** "Infamous crime against nature" is punishable by 30 days in jail and/or $500.

3. **Arkansas:** Oral or anal sex with someone of the same sex is punishable by one year and/or $1000.

4. **Florida:** An "unnatural and lascivious act" is punishable by 60 days in jail and/or $500.

5. **Georgia:** Oral or anal sex are punishable by 20 years in jail.

6. **Idaho:** An "infamous crime against nature" is punishable by life in prison.

7. **Kansas:** Oral or anal sex with someone of the same sex is punishable by 6 months in jail and/or $1000.

8. **Louisiana:** "Unnatural carnal copulation" is punishable by five years in prison and/or $2000.

9. **Maryland:** Oral or anal sex with someone of the same sex is punishable by 10 years in prison and/or $1000.

10. **Massachusetts:** "Sodomy" and "buggery" are punishable offenses.

11. **Michigan:** "Abominable and detestable crimes against nature" are punishable by 15 years in prison or $2500.

12. **Minnesota:** Oral or anal sex are punishable by one year in prison and/or $3000.

13. **Missouri:** Oral or anal sex with someone of the same sex are punishable by one year in prison and $1,000.

14. **North Carolina:** "Crimes against nature" are punishable by 10 years in prison.

15. **Oklahoma:** "Detestable and abominable crimes against nature" with anyone of the same sex are punishable by 10 years in prison.

16. **Rhode Island:** An "abominable and detestable crime against nature" is punishable by 20 years in prison (7 minimum).

17. **South Carolina:** An "abominable crime of buggery" is punishable by five years in prison and/or $500.

18. **Utah:** Oral or anal sex with anyone other than one's spouse is punishable by six months in jail or $299.

19. **Virginia:** Oral or anal sex are punishable by 20 years in prison.

I will resist the efforts of some to obtain government endorsement of homosexuality.

—Ronald Reagan

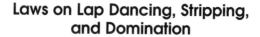

Laws on Lap Dancing, Stripping, and Domination

The prudish nature of politicians has created a climate where stripping, lap dancing, and domination is highly regulated. We've assembled several examples.

1. In several states strip clubs are banned because they are considered to be breaking laws that limit people from engaging

in sexual conduct for money. A Texas law passed in 1998 made it tough in certain areas for strip clubs to exist.

2. One of the first states to enact laws that dealt with lap dancing in particular was Florida. In 1992 their District Court of Appeals held that lap dancing was "lewd" conduct under Section 796.07(2)(a) of the Florida statutes, which prohibited operating a building for purposes of lewdness, warranting revocation of an alcoholic beverage license.

3. While this sort of discrimination is surprising in a place like Florida, known for nude beaches and sexy salsa dancing, it is not too surprising that Nebraska would pass laws outlawing stripping. In 1994 the Nebraska Court of Appeals ruled that "lap dancing" and certain other sexual activity violated a city ordinance that prohibited "lewd, indecent or lascivious" behavior.

4. Canada has had several monumental court cases about lap dancing. One of the first court cases went to trial in 1996. The Ontario Court of Appeals found that it was legally sound to prohibit lap dancing, as there were laws that ban "immoral" performances.

5. Another common way in which strip clubs are limited is through buffer-zone laws. These ordinances limit strip clubs by imposing rules that force clubs to maintain anywhere from a three- to ten-foot separation between patrons and dancers. Prior to a 1977 amendment to the New York Alcoholic Beverage Law prohibiting topless dancing, the ABC Regulation permitted topless dancing " . . . on a stage or platform which is at least 18 inches above the immediate floor level and at least six feet from the nearest patron."

6. Washington State has an ordinance that requires dancers to stay ten feet away from patrons. The ordinance also required

a raised platform for performers at least 18 inches off the floor. The state claimed that this law was created to prohibit the encouragement of prostitution, drug usage, and the sale of drugs in strip clubs.

7. Newport Beach, California, also has buffer laws. They require adult entertainers to perform on a stage at least 18 inches high and to stay at least six feet away from customers. The law also states that adult entertainers are to have no contact with customers and that no tipping is to be allowed.

8. Other cities with buffer laws include Seattle, Amarillo, Phoenix, New York City, Beaumont, Houston, Austin, Indianapolis, and Oklahoma City. Some states such as Idaho are trying to outlaw strip clubs altogether.

9. Professional dominatrixes are also being called into court. Terri-Jean Bedford went to court in 1999 for sex charges. Bedford admits to having tortured and humiliated clients, but that no sexual contact occurred. Her lawyer, Alan Young, told the panel of judges that Bedford, a Toronto resident, charged money to men to help them act out their fantasies, but without bodily fluid exchange and without overt sexual contact. Her home featured theme rooms such as a dungeon, classroom, and nursery. Bedford was found guilty and fined $3,000 for operating a house of prostitution.

In the sex field, you can be totally stupid and still make money.

—Al Goldstein

——◆——

Laws That Regulate Cohabitation or Fornication Between Consenting Adults

These laws involve fornication and/or cohabitation.

1. **Alaska:** Cohabitation is considered a punishable offense.

2. **Arizona:** Cohabitation is punishable by 30 days in jail, and/or a $500 fine.

3. **Florida:** Cohabitation is considered a punishable offense and can be punished by 60 days in jail and/or a $500 fine.

4. **Georgia:** Fornication is illegal and is punishable by one year in jail and/or a $1,000 fine.

5. **Idaho:** Fornication/cohabitation are punishable by 6 months in jail and/or a $300 fine.

6. **Illinois:** Fornication/cohabitation are illegal and punishable by six months in jail and/or a $500 fine.

7. **Massachusetts:** Cohabitation is punishable by three months in jail and/or a $300 fine.

8. **Michigan:** Cohabitation is punishable by one year in jail and/or a $500 fine.

9. **New Mexico:** Cohabitation is a punishable crime.

10. **North Carolina:** Fornication/cohabitation are both punishable by six months in jail and/or a $500 fine.

11. **Rhode Island:** Fornication is punishable by a $10 fine.

12. **South Carolina:** Fornication/cohabitation are punishable by one year in jail and/or a $500 fine.

13. **Utah:** Fornication is punishable by six months in jail and/or a $299 fine.

14. **Vermont:** Fornication is a punishable offense.

15. **Virginia:** Fornication is punishable by a $100 fine.

16. **Washington, DC:** Fornication is considered illegal and is punishable by six months in jail and/or a $300 fine.

17. **West Virginia:** Fornication/cohabitation are both punishable by a $20 minimum fine and six months jail.

18. **Wisconsin:** Fornication is punishable.

*It could be said that the advance of civilization
has not so much moulded modern sexual
behavior, as that sexual behavior has moulded
the shape of civilization.*

—Desmond Morris, *The Naked Ape*

——————◆——————

Age of Consent in the United States

The age of consent is, in all states, a felony matter. Those who engage in sexual relations with a minor can, and will be, charged to the fullest extent of the law under the individual state statutes. While we have researched the age of consent in the different states and the information given in this list is accurate to the best of our knowledge as of Summer, 2000 we are not lawyers and this information should not have any bearing on the choices of the reader. In other words, even though this information is researched, it is by no means a legal document, endorsement, or guarantee. So, to those who would want to or would be dumb enough to actually engage in sexual relations with a minor, you risk your own life in the legal and penal system.

2 States Where the Age of Consent Is 14

Georgia

Hawaii (Persons 15 to 18 may marry with parental consent.)

6 States Where the Age of Consent Is 15

Colorado

Iowa

Maryland

North Dakota

South Carolina

Virginia

30 States Where the Age of Consent Is 16

Alabama (Persons under 14 may marry with parental consent.)

Alaska

Arkansas

Connecticut

Delaware

District of Columbia

Indiana

Kansas

Kentucky

Maine

Massachusetts

Michigan

Minnesota

Montana

Nebraska

Nevada

New Hampshire (Males 14 or over and females 13 or over can marry with parental consent. Marriage laws were enacted in 1907.)

New Jersey

New Mexico

North Carolina (An unmarried female who is between age 12 and 18 may marry the father of her child with parental consent or the con-

North Carolina (*cont.*)

    sent of the director of her local social services in the county in which she resides.)

Ohio

Oklahoma

Oregon (It is also a felony to cause someone under the age of 18 to touch the sex organs of an animal for sexual purposes.)

Pennsylvania (It is also a felony to seduce someone under the age of 18 with a promise of marriage.)

Rhode Island

South Dakota

Utah

Vermont

Washington

West Virginia

5 States Where the Age of Consent Is 17

Illinois

Louisiana

Missouri

New York

Texas

8 States Where the Age of Consent Is 18

Arizona (It is a felony for anyone to have sexual contact with the breast of a girl under age 15.)

California

Florida (It is a felony in Florida to commit sexual interactions, including masturbation, bestiality, and sadomasochism, in front of someone under 16.)

Idaho

Mississippi

Tennessee

Wisconsin (It is also a felony to cause someone under 18 to go into a building, room, vehicle, or any other place with the intent of having sexual relations.)

Wyoming

A man is only as old as the woman he feels.

—Groucho Marx

Legal Definitions of Sexual Terms

So, you think you know erotica from pornography from the merely indecent? Look at it through the eyes of the law:

1. **Hardcore.** According to the courts, hardcore pornography appeals to the "sick and morbid" interests in people, is offensive according to "community standards," and has no redeeming value.

2. **Prurient.** The U.S. Supreme Court has defined as prurient any material that creates lustful thoughts in the viewer.

3. **Erotica.** Like the term "natural" on a box of cereal, the term "erotica" has no legal meaning. It's a matter of individual beliefs.

4. **Pornography.** Like erotica, pornography also has no legal meaning. Decisions of the court are about "obscenity," not about whether or not something is "pornography."

5. **Indecent.** Not conforming to community standards of propriety or modesty.

6. **Obscenity.** The definition of obscenity has changed five times over the last 150 years. The current standard (since 1973) is called the Miller Standard. Something is obscene if (a) the dominant theme appeals to prurient interests and (b) the material is offensive because it affronts contemporary community standards and (c) the material lacks serious liter-

ary, artistic, political, or scientific value. The courts have ruled that obscene material may be regulated by the state under the first amendment.

It'll be a sad day for sexual liberation when the pornography addict has to settle for the real thing.

—Brendan Francis

CHAPTER 5

Internet

Best Sexual Education Sites on the Internet

These sites can teach you silly things about sex—like mrskin.com, who tells you the movies in which your favorite stars have appeared naked—serious business, like the intelligent and far-reaching sexuality.org. School was never this much fun.

- *Safer Sex:* http://www.safesex.com
- *Sex Education for Teens:* http://scarleteen.com
- *The Adult Movie FAQ:* http://www.rame.net/faq/
- *Adult Sexy Web:* http://www.minou.com/adultsexuality.com
- *Fetish Information Exchange:* http://fetishclub.com/exchange
- *Mr. Skin:* http://www.mrskin.com
- *On the Ropes.com:* http://www.ontheropes.com/scripts/start.asp
- *Pam's Guide:* http://www.pamsguide.com
- *The Steel Door:* http://www.steel-door.com/chamber.html
- *Pink Slip:* http://www.scarletters.com/pink
- *Sex Ed 101:* http://www.sexed101.com
- *The Society for Human Sexuality:* http://www.sexuality.org

There's no such thing as safe sex. I really believe that. There may be semi-safe sex, but I don't think you can really say it's safe.

—Barbara Bush

174

Best Fetish Sites

Some are free, some cost to get in, but all are weird! Enter at your own risk.

- *Bondage.com:* http://www.bondage.com

- *Erotic Punishment:* http://www.eroticpunishment.com

- *Fetish Hotel:* http://www.fetishhotel.com

- *Fetish Park:* http://fetishpark.com

- *D/s Kiosk:* http://www.cuffs.com

- *The House of Latex & Bondage:* http://www.latexfetish.com

- *Linda's Foot Fetish:* http://www.dailydosage.com

- *Spider's Torture Web:* http://www.desade.com

- *Laura's Spanking Corner:* http://www.goodkitty.com/spanking/stories/laura/

Is sex dirty? Only if it's done right.

—Woody Allen

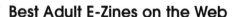

Best Adult E-Zines on the Web

Some free, some cost. We especially recommend the free newsletters are "How to Succeed with Women" and "How to Succeed with Men," which are both written by your authors, who also wrote the books entitled *How to Succeed with Women* and *How to Succeed with Men.*

- *How to Succeed with Women Newsletter:* http://www.howtosucceed-withwomen.com

- *How to Succeed with Men Newsletter:* http://www.howtosucceed-withmen.com

- *Skin Two:* http://www.skintwo.co.uk

- *Adult Video News Magazine:* http://www.avn.com

- *Playboy Magazine:* http://www.playboy.com

- *Penthouse Magazine:* http://www.penthouse.com

- *VaVoom Magazine:* http://www.vavoom.com

- *Genesis Magazine:* http://www.genesismagazine.com

- *Hustler:* http://www.just18.com

- *Adult Stars Magazine:* http://www.adultstarsmag.com

- *Scarlet Letters:* http://www.scarletletters.com

No one ever died from an overdose of pornography.

—J. Money and P. Tucker

◆

Best Gay Sites

- *Gay.com:* http://www.gay.com

- *Absolutely Male:* http://www.absolutelymale.com

- *Badpuppy:* http://www.badpuppy.com

- *Bed Fellow:* http://www.bedfellow.com

- *Boy Zone:* http://www.boyzone.com
- *Chisel Media:* http://www.chisel.com
- *Company Men:* http://www.companymen.com
- *Naked Sword:* http://www.nakedsword.com
- *Planet Stud:* http://www.planetstud.com

> **This sort of thing may be tolerated by the French,
> but we are British—thank God.**
>
> —Lord Montgomery

Hot-Link Sites

Often the best way to cruise the net for sex sites is to let someone else do the browsing for you and to present you with a list of the best. Here are some of the top sex-link resources:

- *Adult Video News Magazine:* http://avn.com
- *Al-4A:* http://www.al4a.com/links.html
- *AltaVisex:* http://www.altavisex.com
- *Carnal Planet:* http://www.carnalplanet.com
- *Eros Find:* http://www.erosfind.com
- *Erotic Desires Top 100:* http://www.eroticdesires.com/top100/
- *Jane's Guide:* http://www.janesguide.com
- *Naughty Linx:* http://www.naughtylinx.com
- *Persian Kitty:* http://www.persiankitty.com

- *Wet Place:* http://www.wetplace.com

- *YouHO!:* http://www.youho.com

*I don't think pornography is very harmful,
but it is terribly, terribly boring.*

—Noël Coward

———◆———

Best Erotic Photography Sites

Some of these are pay, some are free, all have samples.

- *Andrew Blake:* http://www.andrewblake.com

- *Color Climax:* http://www.colorclimax.com

- *Digital Dream Girls:* http://www.ddgirls.com/tour_2/index.html

- *Fresh Photos:* http://www.freshphotos.com

- *Kinky Machine:* http://www.kinkymachine.com

- *Nerve Magazine:* http://www.nerve.com

- *Pixotna:* http://www.pixotna.com

- *Puritan Sex:* http://www.puritansex.com

- *Studio Jorgen:* http://www.studiojorgen.com

- *Suze Randall:* http://www.suzerandall.com

*I feel like a kid in the world's biggest
candy store.*

—Hugh Hefner

———◆———

Best Hardcore Sites

Here are the hard-core sites you might want to check out, in alphbetical order:

- *Club Love:* http://www.clublove.com
- *Cybererotica:* http://www.cybererotica.com
- *Danni's Hard Drive:* http://www.danni.com
- *Kara's Adult Playground:* http://www.karasxxx.com
- *Puritan Sex:* http://www.puritansex.com
- *Private:* http://www.private.com
- *Pure Hardcore:* http://www.purehardcore.com
- *Red Light Asia:* http://www.redlightasia.com
- *Video Secrets:* http://www.videosecrets.com
- *Vivid Video:* http://www.vividvideo.com

Some things are better than sex, some things are worse, but there's nothing exactly like it.

—W. C. Fields

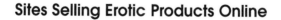

Sites Selling Erotic Products Online

Why buy sex toys or clothes where everyone can stare at you? Online, no one knows what you are into.

- *Erotic books:* Amazon.com: http://www.amazon.com
- *Erotic books:* eroticbooks.com: http://www.eroticbooks.com

- *Sex videos:* Videoage: http://videoage.com
- *Sexual toys:* Sextoyworld: http://www.sextoyworld.com
- *Toys, videos, clothes:* Church Sluts: http://www.churchsluts.com
- *Lingerie:* Fredericks of Hollywood: http://www.fredericks.com
- *Lingerie:* Victoria's Secret: http://www.victoriassecret.com
- *Sex clothes:* Nightwear: http://www.nightwear.com
- *Leather, PVC lingerie, including "plus" sizes:* Leather Butterfly: http://www.leatherbutterfly.com
- *Web-based sexy greeting cards:* Kinky Cards: http://www.kinky cards.com
- *Gay videos, books, toys:* http://www.manshop.com
- *Sex toys, books, video, very woman friendly:* http://www.good vibes.com
- *Sex toys, books, video, very woman friendly and woman-owned:* A Woman's Touch http://www.a-womans-touch.com

Sex—the poor man's polo.

—Clifford Odets

Personal Ads Sites

There are sites all over the Web that want to help you find your mate, no matter your persuasion. Here are some of the biggest:

- *America On-Line Personals:* (all types). http://www.loveataol.com
- *Yahoo Personals (all types):* http://www.personals.yahoo.com

- *Match.com (all types):* http://www.match.com

- *Alt.com (fetish personal ads):* http://www.alt.com

- *Alternative Connections (all alternative sexualities):* http://www.alternativeconnections.com

- *Adult Friend Finder (just sex and swinging):* http://www.adultfriendfinder.com

- *Out Personals (gay):* http://www.outpersonals.com

- *Jail Babes (women in jail):* http://www.jailbabes.com

- *Darquest (men in jail):* http://www.darquest.com

- *Military Babes (military women):* http://www.militarybabes.com

- *Military Men (men in the military):* http://www.militarymen.com

It is better to be unfaithful than to be faithful without wanting to be.

—Brigitte Bardot

CHAPTER 6

Other Cultures

Religious Views on Sexuality

Religion has been the major driving force in determining sexual mores and values. Religion has impacted what is considered obscene and what is considered immoral. Each of the major world religions have a different perspective on sexuality. You can compare and contrast the different belief systems and compare them to your own.

1. Catholicism

Within Catholicism masturbation is a sin. Most forms of birth control are banned. Outside-of-marriage sex is prohibited. The role of sex within a marriage is for procreation. Both Catholic priests and nuns must be celibate.

2. Islam

Some Islamic countries sentence to death those who commit adultery. Thus, relationships outside of marriage are strictly forbidden. Members of Islamic clergy are not required to be celibate.

3. Buddhism

The bases of sexual conduct come down to whether or not the sexual activity will harm another person. If it does not harm or exploit someone then it is permissible. Monks and nuns are required to be celibate.

4. Judaism

The Jewish faith does not require any member of the clergy to be celibate. Sex is seen as something for pleasure as well as procreation inside of marriage. Sex on the Sabbath is considered to be of merit.

5. Hinduism

Part of the struggle for enlightenment for Hindu monks is to practice celibacy. Being free from lust is said to help monks be ego free as well as free from materialistic attachments. For those who are not monks or nuns, sex is restricted for marriage.

6. Protestantism

Clergy members of the Protestant community are not required to take celibacy vows. Sex is viewed as a part of a marriage and is discouraged outside of marriage.

> *I think the essence of Judao/Christian teachings is very similar to* Playboy.
>
> —Hugh Hefner

Foreign-Language Survival Kit

International travel can always be stressful, especially when you do not speak the language. We feel that it is crucial that you be able to communicate when traveling about what is most important . . . sex. Memorize these words and you will be fine in any social situation when traveling. We have listed the English word or phrase first and then the translated variation.

1. Fellatio

Spanish = *mamada*
Italian = *bocchino*
French = *plume*

2. My wife and I would like to make it with you

Spanish = *Mi mujer y yo queremos follar contigo*
Japanese = *Ianai to watashi to issho ni shitai*
Arabic = *Ana ow murati anez ien nik-nak mahbat surng chong wan ha*
French = *Ma femme et moi aimerons la faire avec toi*
German = *Meine Frau und ich wollen es mit Dir treiben*

3. Semen

Spanish = *leche*
Italian = *sburro*
French = *foutre*

4. Anus

German = *Arsch* French = *cul*
Spanish = *culo* Italian = *culo*

5. Vagina

German = *Fotze* Italian = *fica*
Spanish = *cono* French = *con*

6. Orgasm

German = *kommen* Italian = *venire*
Spanish = *correrse* French = *jouir*

7. To have an erection

German = *einen ständer haben*
Spanish = *pararse*
Italian = *rizzarsi*
French = *bander*

8. I am a masochist; I need a sadist

Spanish = *Soy masoquista y, busco a un sadico(a)*
Japanese = *Watashi wa mazohisuto desu, sadisto ga hoshii*
Arabic = *Ana beta* masochist, ana awez sádut
French = *Je sui un masochiste; j'ai besoin d'um sadiste*
German = *Ich bin ein Masochist, ich brauche einen Sadist*

9. Prostitute

German = *Hure* Italian = *puttana*
Spanish = *puta* French = *putain*

10. Condom

German = *Gummi*   Italian = *guanto*
Spanish = *goma*   French = *capote anglaise*

11. Penis

German = *Schwanz*   Italian = *cazzo*
Spanish = *carajo*   French = *bite*

12. Masturbate

German = *abwichsen*   Italian = *farsi una sega*
Spanish = *hacer puñetas*   French = *se branter*

**Sex is like money—very nice to have
but vulgar to talk about.**

—Tonia Berg

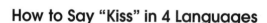

How to Say "Kiss" in 4 Languages

1. German

Kuss, a kiss

Abschiedskuss (AP-sheets-kus), farewell kiss

Versöhnungskuss (fer-SEUN-ungs-kus), a make-up kiss

2. Spanish

Beso (BEy-so), a kiss

Besame (bey-sa-may) "kiss me"

3. French

Embrasse-mo (ahm-BRAHS-mwah), polite form, "kiss me"

Baise-moi (beh-mwah), vulgar form of "kiss me"

4. Italian

Il bàcio (ell-BOT-show), a kiss

> *Never delay kissing a pretty girl of opening a bottle of whiskey.*
>
> —Ernest Hemingway

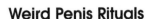

Weird Penis Rituals

We call this list "weird penis rituals" to distinguish it from normal, nonweird penis rituals—meaning ones that Westerners are used to, such as male infant circumcision. Hey, that's perfectly normal, right?

- Polynesians cut the foreskin lengthwise at puberty.

- Some African tribes have practiced semi-castration—the removal of one testicle.

- Australian Aborigines of the Walibri clan greet neighboring tribes during ceremonies by shaking penises, rather than hands.

- The Aborigines also slit the penis so it could be flattened to resemble that of the kangaroo.

- In Borneo the Dayak tribe inserted a metal rod with balls on its ends across the top of the penis.

- Many tribes in Africa practice ritual circumcision, including the Xhosa, the tribe of Nelson Mandela. He speaks in his autobiography about his initiation, as a teenager, when the *Ingcibi*, or circumcision expert, cut off his foreskin with an *assegai*, or knife. The initiate then yells, "*Ndiyindoda!*" ("I am a man!")

- In some tribes in Africa birth control is performed through what is known colloquially as a "whistle cock." A slit is made across the urethra just in front of the scrotum, so the semen flows out through the slit, rather than into the woman's vagina.

- In Burma men of the Peguans tribe would insert small bells under the skin of the penis.

There's nothing more fun than a man.

—Dorothy Parker

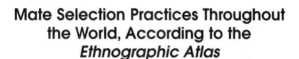

Mate Selection Practices Throughout the World, According to the *Ethnographic Atlas*

1. Twenty-one percent of women worldwide have their partner chosen for them by their parents, and there's nothing they can do about it.

2. Thirteen percent of men worldwide have their partner chosen for them by their parents, and there's nothing they can do about it.

3. Seventeen percent of women live in societies where some marriages are arranged, and others are based on individual choices.

4. Eighteen percent of men live in such societies.

5. Three percent of men and three percent of women live in societies where many people, such as parents and family members, must agree on mates.

6. Twenty-nine percent of women can select their own mate, with social approval "highly desirable."

7. Nineteen percent of men can select their own mate, with social approval "highly desirable."

8. Eight percent of women live in societies where they can select their mates with no social approval necessary.

9. Thirty-one percent of men live in such societies.

Every woman should marry—and no man.

—Benhamin Disraeli

———◆———

Wedding and Wedding Night Rituals

- In some places in Ecuador the husband can return the bride to her family if he determines that she is not a virgin.

- In some places in Colombia, when the newly married couple has sex for the first time the bride's mother watches.

- In some African tribes that practice "infibulation" (the sewing shut of a girl's vagina, leaving only enough of an opening for urine and menstrual fluid to escape), the act of cutting the vagina back open ("defibulation") is done by the husband or a midwife after marriage.

- Among the Marind-anim people of New Guinea, a bride has sex with all the men in her husband's clan in a kind of marriage ceremony called *Otiv Bombari*. This ceremony also takes place after the birth of a child. The women are reported not to like this ritual very much.

- In the Bohindu tribe in Africa the husband has to remain celibate until his new wife is pregnant by another man.

- Some Hindu, South American, and Indonesian cultures believe that virginity can have magical powers over men. In these societies the hymens of baby girls are broken, so the bride's virginity will not exact dangerous power over the groom.

- In many Western cultures, rice or some other grain is thrown on newlyweds to symbolize (and even ensure) fertility.

- In the Darmstadt district of Germany, young unmarried women surround the bride at the wedding and must defend her from the matrons, who seek to tear off her bridal wreath and her shoes, as symbols of her coming loss of virginity.

- The "right of first night," or *jus primae noctis*, refers to the rumored right of the tribal headman or king to have sex with any bride before the husband does. This ritual was mentioned in the Sumerian *Epic of Gilgamesh*, a story that is about 5,000 years old. In it the emperor Gilgamesh "leaves no wife to the husband," instead demanding she be sent to him before going to her marriage bed.

- In the Tanzanian Zaramo tribe, two women watch as the newlyweds make love for the first time to assess both the woman and the man. To decide if the woman is a virgin, they watch for blood and to see how easy she is to penetrate. The groom is judged by the amount and thickness of his semen.

- In some areas of Latvia, Lithuania, and Poland the bride is forced with a stick to enter the wedding chamber and to lie on the wedding bed.

- The Amhara people of Ethiopia place great emphasis on the first coupling of a newlywed couple. Late in the day of the wedding, the bride and the groom ignore each other and the guests ignore them both, except to joke about the coming "battle." At the appointed time they go into the marriage hut, where they disrobe and get into bed, staying as far from each other as possible. After several minutes the man leaps upon the woman without warning. She has been instructed to fight him off. He must show he has the power to take what he wants, and she must show that she is no weakling. In time, they consummate their marriage. Meanwhile, the guests have been listening to all this from outside the hut. They may place bets on the outcome of the struggle and on whether or not the bride is a virgin.

After the sex act, a cloth that had been placed under the bride is taken by the matron of honor directly to the best man. If it is appropriately bloody (proving the bride's virginity), he puts it on his head with a cap over it, and everybody dances. The cloth is then taken to the parents of the bride, who wrap the dowry in it and give it back.

Lie still and think of England.

—Old advice to a British bride
on her wedding night

Sexual Festivals

Traditional and historical cultures seemed to believe in the importance of having festivals or carnivals where they could "let it all hang out," then return to the strictures of normal society for yet another year.

- In Santali, India, the Sohrae harvest festival is celebrated for three to six days. During it there is much drinking and merriment and a general relaxation of social and sexual mores—married couples engage in extramarital relations, and newlyweds have liaisons with former lovers.

- During Phoenician harvest festivals, a woman could choose either to have sex with a stranger or shave her head as a sign of mourning for the sacrifice of the harvest god—either choice was completely acceptable.

- Aphrodite's birthday was celebrated with a ritual bath and orgy.

- As part of the funeral rites in some parts of the Melanesian Islands, married women have sex with men and boys after the burial.

- When men of the Turkhana tribe in Africa are circumcised, they may have sex with any woman they choose.

- In medieval Cologne, Germany, during Carnival, masked and drunken revelers would have orgies in public dance halls.

- In ancient Greek and Roman times, Bacchanalian festivals involved carrying giant representations of the male phallus through the streets, garlanded with flowers. Wild dances were held that routinely led to wild orgies.

- In Hawaii, when a chief died there were several days of excess, lawlessness, and sexual license and public expression. Law and order did not return until the new chief was installed into office.

- Among the Kiwai of coastal Papua-New Guinea, one fertility ritual consisted of several nights of unrestricted sexual congress, during which the sperm of the men was collected from the women and put in a container, along with other ingredients, where it could be used on anything that needed increased fertility.

- In one tribe in New Guinea, this celebration took place, at least up to the early 1900s: Young men who were to be initiated were, as part of the ceremony, sent into the woods to have sex with any woman of their choosing. The young man would bring a broken tree branch back with him to symbolize his success. There would be several days of much sexual congress, culminating in a ritual in which a young man and woman would have sex in a great wooden hut. The others would then sacrifice these two by pulling the wooden hut down on them, killing them. They were then cut up and roasted as a feast for the tribe.

If all the young ladies who attended the Yale promenade dance were laid end to end, no one would be the least surprised.

—Dorothy Parker

———◆———

How to Say "I Love You"

Love is the international language, right? Then you'd better know how to say "I love you" no matter where you go.

Afrikaans	*Ek het jou lief*
Arabic	*Ana Ba-heb-bak*
Bengali	*Ami tomay bhalobashi*
Bulgarian	*Ahs Obichum te*
Cantonese	*Ngo oi lei*
Chinese	*Wo aì ni*
Czech	*Miluji te*
Danish	*Jeg elsker dig*
Dutch	*Ik hou van jou*
French	*Je t'aime*
German	*Ich liebe Dich*
Hmong	*Kuv hlub koj*
Hungarian	*Szeretlek*
Indonesian	*Saja kasih saudari*
Japanese	*Aishiteru*
Korean	*Nanun niga joa*
Polish	*Ja cie kocham*
Russian	*Ya vas lyublyu*
Samoan	*Oute alofa ia te oe*
Spanish	*Te amo*
Swedish	*Jag älskar dig*
Thai	*Phom rak khun*
Vietnamese	*Toi yeu em*

Immature love says: "I love you because I need you." Mature love says: "I need you because I love you."

—Erich Fromm

CHAPTER 7

Celebrity Sex

17 Masturbation Scenes from Popular Films

1. Body Double
Melanie Griffith plays a porn star in this film who is famous for her masturbation scenes.

2. American Beauty
Kevin Spacey masturbates twice in this film, once while in the shower and later while in his bed while his wife is asleep.

3. The Bad Lieutenant
Harvey Keitel plays a police lieutenant in this controversial film. In one scene he masturbates while watching two teen-aged girls expose themselves to him in their car.

4. Single White Female
The ever-popular Jennifer Jason Leigh is seen masturbating alone in her room in this 1992 movie.

5. Law of Desire
Antonio Banderas is seen masturbating in this movie while watching horror movies.

6. The Blue Lagoon
In this film starring Brooke Shields, Chris Atkins is caught masturbating by Shields.

7. Body of Evidence
The ever-popular sex symbol Madonna masturbates while Wilhem Dafoe watches with hunger.

8. Tommy Boy

David Spade is seen masturbating as he watches a sexy naked woman swim in a swimming pool.

9. 9-1/2 Weeks

Sex symbol Kim Bassinger masturbates while watching a slide show in this very sexy 1986 controversial film.

10. The Basketball Diaries

Leonardo di Caprio stars in this movie and is seen playing with himself on the roof of his New York apartment building.

11. Even Cowgirls Get the Blues

Uma Thurman is seen masturbating in her car on the side of a highway.

12. Tie Me Up! Tie Me Down!

Victoria Abril masturbates several times in this film. First she is seen masturbating while watching pornography on TV. She is later seen masturbating with a dildo.

13. Being There

In this 1979 Peter Sellers movie, Shirley MacLaine masturbates while the unusual star of the movie (Chance) watches TV.

14. Boogie Nights

Mark Wahlberg plays a character who is offered money to masturbate. He does it for $10.

15. Extra-Marital

Sex queen Traci Lords is seen masturbating in bed while listening to another couple make love.

16. Naked Gun 33-1/3

There is a brief scene in which Leslie Nielson masturbates in a sperm donation clinic.

17. Gia

This HBO movie stars Angelina Jolie. In one scene she is seen wearing mens' underwear and touching herself.

> **Don't knock masturbation. It's sex with someone I love.**
>
> —From *Annie Hall*

———◆———

Top 10 Hottest Women

In a landmark research study conducted by the Louis & Copeland think tank, men across the United States admitted which women they most frequently fantasized about. The findings to this study are shocking. Here they are:

1. Pamela Anderson Lee
2. Demi Moore
3. Shania Twain
4. Cindy Crawford
5. Carmen Electra
6. Jennifer Lopez
7. Tyra Banks
8. Salma Hayek
9. Jennifer Aniston
10. Heather Locklear

*Sex is one of nine reasons for reincarnation . . .
The other eight are unimportant.*

—Henry Miller, *Big Sur and the Oranges
of Hieronymus Bosch*

———◆———

Elvis Presley: Sex Facts, Rumors, and Factoids

Elvis literally is the king of sex. He revolutionized sexuality in the media and the notion of sexual expression. Elvis was one of most loved performers of his day. We've all heard the rumors of Elvis sightings. While they seem crazy, he was and still is such a legend that people want to believe he is still alive, still available to touch and to inspire. Here is a smattering of his many sexual experiences and relationships throughout his life.

1. Elvis was born in 1935 and died, in 1977 at age 42, from a drug overdose.

2. Though he was an international star, Elvis was a gun freak, drug addict, and womanizer.

3. Some biographers claim that Elvis slept with more than 1,000 women during his lifetime.

4. Sexual nicknames for the King include, "Elvis the Pelvis" and "Sir Swivel Hips."

5. The King was feared by the media and by the conservative faction of America. Billy Graham mentioned that he did not want his daughter to meet Elvis.

6. Elvis was the highest paid musician of all time. It is estimated that he grossed over $1 billion in his lifetime.

7. Elvis starred in 23 films and stopped making them in 1970.

8. It is rumored that he had a 14-year affair with Virginia Sullivan, whom he met when she was a cashier in a movie theater. The affair supposedly took place from 1953 until 1967.

9. Elvis first had an affair with Dixie Lock in 1954, when he was 19, she was 15. They met at a roller rink.

10. Before Elvis dated Priscilla he was actively involved with 16-year-old Margit Buergin. She was a typist who lived in Germany.

11. Elvis first met Anita Wood when she was 19 and hosting a teen music TV show in Memphis. They dated from 1957 until 1962.

12. Biographers claim that an unnamed woman spent the weekend with the King in Florida. The woman nearly died in the middle of the night. She and Elvis drank large quantities of cough syrup containing narcotics. She was rushed to the hospital and survived.

13. Elvis first met Priscilla Beaulieu when he was in Germany with the army in 1959. Beaulieu was 14 at the time. She was gorgeous, but the daughter of an army captain. Soon they began spending every free moment together. He would even send a driver to pick her up at school. She went to live with Elvis after she turned 16.

14. Elvis married Priscilla in 1967 upon the request of Beaulieu's father.

15. He divorced Priscilla in 1973. She was awarded $2 million in the final divorce settlement.

16. Elvis lusted after Ann-Margaret. They dated for a brief period, and it is said that they were in love.

17. Elvis briefly dated Debra Paget, the co-star of *Love Me Tender*. She claims that he asked her to marry him, but she refused.

18. After dating Paget, it is rumored that Elvis dated Natalie Wood.

19. He had a brief fling with Debra Walley in 1966. She was the costar of the movie *Spinout*.

20. It is rumored that the King liked petite women with shapely legs and buttocks. He was not a breast man.

21. Many biographers claim that Elvis had a kinky side to him. Supposedly, he enjoyed videotaping women when he had sex with them.

22. It is rumored that he loved mirrored ceilings so he could watch himself while he was doing "it." Furthermore, it is said that many of the bedrooms in his home had one-way mirrors in them so he could watch guests undress and have sex.

23. On several occasions the King was said to have hired two or three prostitutes to have sex with each other while he watched and enjoyed solo sex.

24. Elvis managed to steal Barbara Leigh from MGM president James Aubrey. The affair took place while he was married to Priscilla. Leigh finally left Elvis when she realized he had no plans of divorcing or leaving Priscilla.

25. It is rumored that Nancy Sinatra was an Elvis fan. Though they never slept together, they did engage in several long and juicy kisses.

26. Elvis had an affair with Tuesday Weld.

27. Some psychologists claim that he was attracted to young and inexperienced women because he felt insecure about his lovemaking skills.

28. In 1972 Elvis began divorce negotiations with Priscilla. During the divorce proceedings he met Linda Thompson. She was Miss Tennessee at the time and still a virgin. They dated off and on for nearly four years. Linda Thompson is now married to Bruce Jenner.

29. When Ginger Alden was 20 she moved in with Elvis. Elvis proposed to Alden in 1977 and gave her a $70,000 engagement ring. He never married Alden. He died seven months after proposing.

30. After his death several women claimed to have made love to his ghost.

Look at the typical American family scene: Man walking around farting! Woman walking around scratching! Kids going around hollering, hey man, fuck that.

—Elvis Presley

---◆---

Phallic Kings: 20 Famous Men Rumored to Have Large Penises

1. Warren Beatty (actor)

2. Sean Cassidy (musician)

3. Wilt Chamberlain (basketball player)

4. Charlie Chaplin (actor)

5. Sean Connery (actor)

6. Gary Cooper (actor)

7. Eddie Fisher (actor)

8. Cary Grant (actor)

9. Jimi Hendrix (musician)

10. Rock Hudson (actor)

11. Lyndon Baines Johnson (president)

12. David Letterman (TV show host)

13. Jack London (writer)

14. Ron Louis and David Copeland (writers)

15. Dean Martin (singer)

16. Steve Martin (comedian)

17. Jim Nabors (actor/singer)

18. Arnold Schwartzeneggar (actor)

19. Frank Sinatra (singer)

20. Chuck Yeager (astronaut)

An erection at will is the moral equivalent of a valid credit card.

—Alex Comfort

Actors Who Have Appeared Naked on the Silver Screen

Here is your opportunity to see some of Hollywood's sexiest actors naked. Some of these well-known celebrities were in sleazy films before they hit the big time, and some appeared naked in the name of art. If you love nude men, these movies are for you.

1. Jan-Michael Vincent in *Buster and Billie* (1974)

2. Spalding Gray in *The Farmer's Daughter* (1975)

3. Sylvestor Stallone in *A Party at Kitty's* (1975)

4. Dennis Hopper in *Tracks* (1976)

5. Gerard Depardieu in *1900* (1977)

6. Peter Firth in *Equis* (1977)

7. Richard Gere in *American Gigolo* (1977)

8. Eric Stoltz in *Haunted Summer* (1988)

9. John Malkovich in *Sheltering Sky* (1990)

10. Jaye Davidson in *Crying Game* (1992)

11. Tim Robbins in *The Player* (1992)

12. Harvey Keitel in *Bad Lieutenant* (1992)

13. James Woods in *In the Curse of the Starving Class* (1995)

*Full frontal nudity . . . has now become accepted
by every branch of the theatrical profession
with the possible exception of lady
accordion players.*

—Dennis Norden

———◆———

Hollywood Couples Rumored to Have Had Sex on the Silver Screen

Our sources claim that these couples really had sex while filming the following movies. Could it be true?

1. Marlon Brando and Maria Schneider (1973) in *Last Tango in Paris*

2. Donald Sutherland and Julie Christie (1973) in *Don't Look Now*

3. Jack Nicholson and Jessica Lange (1981) in *The Postman Always Rings Twice*

4. Bruce Dern and Maud Adams (1981) in *Tattoo*

5. Mickey Rourke and Lisa Bonet (1987) in *Angel Heart*

6. Mickey Rourke and Carre Otis (1990) in *Wild Orchid*

7. Alec Baldwin and Kim Bassinger (1993) in *The Getaway*

*A man in love is incomplete until he is married.
Then he's finished.*

— Zsa Zsa Gabor (1960)

---◆---

Notable Films with Bisexual
or Gay Characters

1. ***The Vampire Lovers*** (1970), directed by Roy Ward Baker

   This movie is part of a long line of unbelievable horror films that have sexual motifs. The story is about a young woman left alone in a mansion by her wealthy mother. In the absence of the mother she seduces the other daughters and drains their blood.

2. ***Dog Day Afternoon*** (1975), directed by Sidney Lumet

   This movie is based on a true story. Al Pachino plays a bisexual who robs a bank to pay for his lover's sex-change operation.

3. ***The Hunger*** (1993), directed by Tony Scott

   This movie is another vampire story with bisexual characters. This time the story is about one vampire bisexual's search for a new lover. The movie features a hot sex scene between Susan Sarandon and Catherine Deneuve. David Bowie also has a starring role.

4. ***The Hotel New Hampshire*** (1984), directed by Tony Richardson

   This movie included a love scene between Nastassja Kinski and Jodie Foster.

206

5. **Beyond Therapy** (1986), directed by Robert Altman

This offbeat comedy starred Jeff Goldblum as a bisexual and examined his relationship with his therapist, Glenda Jackson.

6. **Henry and June** (1990), directed by Phillip Kaufman

In this movie, based on the life of Henry Miller and Anaïs Nin, the character of Nin is played by Marie De Medeiros. She seeks out sexual experiences with both men and women and shows the struggles in her sexual identity through her journals and confessions.

7. **Lost Language of Cranes** (1991), directed by Nigel Finch

This movie was made in the United Kingdom and is based on a novel by David Leavitt. The movie is about a father and son who come out to each other.

8. **The Crying Game** (1992), directed by Neil Jordan

A man explores homosexual love, even though he considers himself straight.

9. **Basic Instinct** (1992), directed by Paul Verhoeven

Sharon Stone and Michael Douglas starred in this film. All of the villains in this movie are either bisexuals or lesbians.

10. **Savage Nights** (1993), directed by Cyril Collard

This movie was written, directed, and starred Cyril Collard. The story is about a bisexual man who has HIV, but makes no attempts to tell any of his lovers. The movie won four Caesar awards in France a few days after Collard's death from AIDS.

11. **Even Cowgirls Get the Blues,** (1993), directed by Gus van Sant

This film, based on a Tom Robbins novel, features Uma Thurman as a bisexual character who becomes a gypsy traveling in search of love.

12. **Wilde** (1998), directed by Brian Gilbert

This has been called the best Oscar Wilde film made. The movie shows his life and the many lovers he had during his life. The film also shows how the legal system treated Wilde for being homosexual and how he struggled for public support.

Eroticism is the magic of vitality, expressed mainly through the awakening of sexual power.

—R. A. Schwaller de Lubicz

CHAPTER 8

Psychology
of Sex

Famous Sex Surveys

There have been many groundbreaking sex surveys that have forever changed the face of sex research. The types of surveys show how far sex research has come in its 50-year history. Social changes as well as political changes can be seen in the type of research as well as the scope of research. Many of these studies have influenced legislation as well as common acceptance of various forms of sexuality. Some of these studies are even humorous.

1. The Kinsey Report

Kinsey and his colleagues interviewed 5,300 men and 5,940 women from 1938 to 1949. His goal was to interview over 100,000 people. He has remained a controversial figure in the field of sex research because some question the sampling methods of his research. Dr. Kinsey broke ground with his research, however, and did one of the largest studies of its kind during his time.

2. Masters and Johnson

Masters and Johnson were pioneers of sex research. They focused on the physiology of sexual response in men and women and did research in laboratories across the country.

William Masters began his research in 1954. At that time no one had ever done laboratory studies of sexual behavior. Masters had to develop his own research techniques. He started his research by interviewing 118 female prostitutes and 27 male prostitutes. At the same time he began to invent instruments to measure sexual responses.

Masters decided that the best form of research would be to have people from the general public engage in sexual behaviors and then observe and measure the responses. He sought out volunteers in medical school and in his community. Subjects were paid, and some female volunteers brought their husbands along. Initially 694 participated in the research. This included men from age 21 to 89 and women from age 18 to 78. He also had 276 couples participate.

3. Psychology Today

The magazine included a 100-item questionnaire in their magazine. They received over 20,000 responses.

4. The McCall's Survey

McCall's magazine did a survey in 1979. More than 20,000 women returned the surveys. Of those who responded nearly 82 percent were married.

5. The Kanter and Zelnick Survey

Melvin Zelnik and John Kanter conducted a study in 1971. Their research included interviewing 4,611 young women between the ages of 15 and 19. The data were useful because they looked at differences in sexual behavior and attitudes of black versus white women.

6. The National AIDS Behavioral Survey

The Centers for Disease Control undertook this project with the intention of understanding the number of people who might be infected with HIV. They collected data from 1990 to 1991 and interviewed over 10,000 adults. Their research was done by randomly dialing telephones to obtain a random sample. They had a 70 percent response rate.

7. African American and Hispanic Youth

Anne Norris and Kathleen Ford conducted a study of the sexual behavior of both Hispanic and African Youth in 1991. Their sample size was quite small. They interviewed 34 African American males and females and 30 Hispanic males and females.

8. Sexuality in Middle and Later Life

Stephen Weiler and Linda George from Duke University conducted one of the only research studies of sexuality in middle-aged and elderly people. Their research utilized local people. They ended up with 278 participants, all of whom were married.

However, they conducted their study at four time periods (1969, 1971, 1973, and 1975).

Weiler and George showed that there was very little decrease in sexual activity over time.

9. Sexual Behavior in France

To deal with the AIDS crisis, a team of French researchers conducted a major sex survey in 1992. They conducted interviews on the telephone followed by letter. The response rate was 76 percent. They interviewed over 20,000 adults between the ages of 18 and 69. The survey looked at how many people had multiple sexual partners (men 13 percent, women 6 percent).

10. The Hite Report

Shere Hite began her research in 1972. She sent out questionnaires to women on the mailing lists of women's groups such as the National Organization of Women. Her research was done with less than 2,000 questionnaires and was published in 1976 as *The Hite Report*. She received widespread criticism, claiming that her work was not a true representation of American women. She also received criticism for the feminist conclusions she drew from the results.

11. National Opinion Research Center

Edward Laumann, distinguished sociologist and researcher at the University of Chicago, headed a team of 220 researchers who set out in 1987 to examine sexual patterns as a way to combat the spread of AIDS. They compiled nearly 3,500 interviews of select men and women between 18 and 59. He had originally wanted to interview over 20,000 people. Famous prude Jesse Helms headed the fight to withdraw government support in 1991. Private organizations contributed monies so that the initial research phase could be completed.

12. Research on Swingers

Gilbert Bartell, anthropologist, did a participant-observer study in 1970 of couples who are swingers. He and his wife contacted swingers by responding to ads in newspapers and sex magazines. He and his wife also attending swinging parties and conventions. He did not tell anyone that he was doing research, but simply that he and his wife wanted to know more about the swinging lifestyle. His research was not statistical significance, but it was controversial.

I don't see much of Alfred any more since he got so interested in sex.

—Mrs. Alfred Kinsey

Men's Top 10 Most Popular Sexual Dreams

We all dream. In dreams we can experience the desires we want but are afraid to express. We can do unspeakable acts without any repercussions. In dreams we can find solace in desires that are nonsensical. Men's sexual dreams provide insight into what they're really thinking when left to their own devices (no pun intended). We have found the most popular dreams and ranked them in order of popularity.

1. An available and eager woman (or a group of available women). This is the most popular male sexual dream.

2. An available and eager woman. Yes, the number-one sexual dream is so prevalent we thought you needed to read it twice.

3. Sex in public. This dream pales in its popularity to an available woman and presupposes that the woman is first available and eager.

4. Erotic and sensual interactions. This type of dream involves massage, kissing, and lots of foreplay.

5. Famous women (need we say more).

6. Kinky and taboo sex. This includes domination, submission, and more.

7. Being seduced by an older woman.

8. Sexy women teasing and taunting a man, but not actually having sex.

9. Being a male stripper and being approached by several women at once and refusing to have sex with them.

10. Homosexual sex.

Men frequently fantasize about fucking a nun, a nurse, or indeed a policewoman, and when I had my house in New York, I had regular johns who would ask for girls in these various disguises.

—Xaviera Hollander

———◆———

7 Sexual Activities Once Considered Mental Illnesses

1. Exhibitionism

The desire to display one's genitalia to the world was once considered a sign of a mental illness.

2. Sexual Sadism

Those who desired to explore sexual sadism (that is, deriving sexual pleasure through inflicting pain upon their partners) were seen as mentally ill and often thought to have with criminal leanings. Sadism was said to be linked to overaggressive tendencies.

3. Sexual Masochism

The sexual desire to be hurt in some manner includes being beaten, whipped, spanked or other masochistic desire. Women who were masochistic were thought to suffer from hysteria.

4. Masturbation

We all know the evils of masturbation. This act has historically been linked to several mental illnesses and even to being possessed by the devil. Early psychologists thought that masturbation led to antisocial behaviors and could even damage the psyche. In the 1800s some demonologists recommended that those who were caught masturbating be castrated. (See the other lists in this book about masturbation for more on this important topic.)

5. Voyeurism

The act of observing strangers naked or having sex has been seen as a sign of a mental illness. While being a "peeping tom" is clearly an illegal activity if done by looking into people's windows or other acts that invade someone's privacy, the desire to do so is clearly not a sign of mental illness or criminal behavior.

6. Cross-dressing

Cross-dressers in the late 1800s were put with the criminally insane. The cross-dressing man or woman was perverted and was unfit to be in public. Cross-dressing was associated with several mental illnesses.

7. Homosexuality

At various stages of history homosexuality was linked to mental illness and criminal activity. As we know, many religious fanatics to this day still see homosexuality as immoral and improper. However, throughout history it has also been treated as a mental illness. In the 1920s homosexuals were given electroshock therapy to cure this "disease." At other times people claimed that they could "deprogram" homosexuals. In 1973 the American Psychiatric Association dropped homosexuality from its list of mental disorders.

There are special conditions, both physical and moral, which dispose to insanity; in women, menstruation with its irregularities, childbirth, and the changes of life are potent influences.

—T. C. Allbutt, *A System of Medicine* (1899)

---◆---

7 Types of Love Relationships

There are many ways to love. Our customary tradition is serial monogamy, whereby there is only one sexual relationship at a time. However, there are other ways to look at love relationships. Against popular opinion, here they are:

1. **Monogamy:** Being committed to one male or one female

2. **Polygyny (or polygimy):** Being married to more than one female

3. **Polyandry:** Being married to more than one male

4. **Polyamory:** Having numerous lovers at one time

5. **Sororal polygyny:** A man marrying several sisters from the same family

6. **Serial monogamy:** Having a series of monogamous relationships

7. **Celibacy:** Having sex with no one. You can be celibate alone, or with a number of people at once. It's all pretty much the same.

There is no remedy for love but to love more.

—Henry David Thoreau

Sex Statistics: The Horrible Truth

1. Researchers claim that 9 percent of college students have engaged in golden showers.

2. The World Health Organization claims that over 100,000 acts of sexual intercourse happen daily.

3. Around 100 calories are burned during intercourse.

4. Erotic asphyxiation is said to cause over 1,000 deaths each year.

5. A 25-year study of Catholic priests showed that over 50 percent break their vow of celibacy.

6. A University of Chicago poll found that American adults have sex an average of 57 times per year.

7. In 1990 the world kissing record was set by Alfred Wolfram. He kissed 8,001 women in eight hours. That equates to kissing a different woman every six seconds.

8. Seventy percent of men feel that being single is easier than being married.

9. According to Harlequin Enterprises, the famed publisher of romance novels, 46 percent of women feel that a good night's sleep is better than sex.

10. A recent *Glamour* magazine poll showed that 12 percent of women have posed nude for a photo.

11. Forty-five percent of men wish their partner had larger breasts.

12. A 1998 *Details* magazine poll showed that 14 percent of women fantasized about Brad Pitt while having intercourse.

13. Most men thrust 60 to 120 times during intercourse.

Sex appeal is fifty percent what you've got and fifty percent what other people think you've got.

—Sophia Loren

Sexual Phobias

Many people have phobias, or specific fears. They are common psychological phenomena. Freud began writing about phobias in the late 1800s and explored their causes and cures. His research may be interesting to those wanting to wade through his research papers, but to most of us the juicy weird phobias are what are most interesting. We have created a list of strange and unusual phobias for your enjoyment.

Phobia	Source of Fear
1. **Anal-castration anxiety**	Fear of toilets and/or defecation
2. **Androphobia**	Fear of men
3. **Anuptaphobia**	Fear of being unmarried
4. **Aulophobia**	Fear of phallic-looking musical instruments
5. **Bromidrosiphobia**	Fear of body smells
6. **Coitophobia**	Fear of sexual intercourse
7. **Cypridophobia**	Fear of getting an STD
8. **Enosiophobia**	Fear of committing a sexual sin
9. **Eurotophobia**	Fear of female genitalia
10. **Gamophobia**	Fear of marriage
11. **Gynophobia**	Fear of women
12. **Haptephobia**	Fear of being touched
13. **Hedenophobia**	Fear of experiencing sexual pleasure
14. **Parthenophobia**	Fear of virgins and/or young girls
15. **Penetration phobia**	Fear of sexual penetration
16. **Phallophobia**	Fear of the penis (especially erect)
17. **Procophobia**	Fear of rectal exams and anal touch
18. **Scataphobia**	Fear of defecation and scat (i.e., excrement)
19. **Scoptophobia**	Fear of being seen naked
20. **Sexophobia**	Fear of anything related to sex
21. **Spermatophobia**	Fear of sperm
22. **Teratophobia**	Fear of offspring being monsters or defective

To be carnally minded is death.

—Romans 8:6

◆

Origins of Sexual Words

Because inquiring minds want to know. . . .

Ass. Ass came from the Anglo-Saxon *arse,* which is still getting good use in Britain today. In Anglo-Saxon times it was not considered impolite; now arse, and its American equivalent, ass, are a little off-color.

Fuck. It's not clear what the origins of fuck are, though the word seems always to have been "dirty." It is probably related to the Latin *pungere,* the French *foutre,* and the German *ficken,* all of which mean "to beat or strike," with a secondary meaning of "to copulate."

Masochism. Leopold von Sacher-Masoch (1836–1895) was an Austrian lawyer and writer who wrote the classic sado-masochist novel, *Venus in Furs.* Masochism is named after him, as he was famous for his desires for pain and humiliation. German neurologist Krafft-Ebin (1840–1902) coined the word that is still used.

Obscenity. From the Latin, meaning "dirty" or "containing filth or excrement."

Onanism. Onanism is an out-of-fashion word for masturbation. It comes from Onan, son of Judah (Genesis 38:9). It is also another word for the withdrawal method of birth control. The word first came into use in the 1740s.

Orgasm. From the Greek, "to swell with wetness."

Penis. Penis is a Latin word, as you might expect. It means "tail." Strangely enough, penis was slang in ancient Rome, and now it's the right and proper word to use. A paintbrush was called a *penicillus* because it looked like a tail; now pencils and penises have more in common than you might have thought.

Pornography. From the Greek, literally "the writing of or about prostitutes."

Sadism. Named for the Marquis de Sade (1740–1814), a French writer who wrote such books as *The 120 Days of Sodom* and *Justine*, in which sexual torture and humiliation were continuous themes.

Vagina. Once again, a Latin word. It originally meant "scabbard" or "sheath."

Venereal. Both this word and "venery" (indulgence in or pursuit of sexual activity) are from the Latin, handed down from Venus (or Veneris), the goddess of love.

Whoever named it necking was a poor judge of anatomy.

—Groucho Marx

———◆———

Current Sex Myths

1. **Alcohol is a sexual stimulant.** Alcohol is a depressant and actually inhibits sexual functioning. It does lower sexual inhibitions, however, making people more likely to say "yes" to sex.

2. **Castration destroys the sex drive.** This is not true in all cases. Testosterone is produced not only by the testicles, but by other organs as well. Men who are sterilized can still have sex drive and erections.

3. **Sterilization in women destroys the sex drive.** It does not.

4. Menopause ends a woman's sex life. Menopause ends a woman's ability to get pregnant, but does not end her desire to have sex—sometimes it even increases.

5. **Hysterectomy ends a woman's sex life.** This is not true. A woman's desire levels may change, but a healthy sex life is quite possible for women after hysterectomy.

6. **There is safe and predictable time in a woman's menstrual cycle when she can't get pregnant.** There are times in a woman's cycle when she is less likely to get pregnant, but most doctors agree there is no absolutely "safe" time.

7. **Most prostitutes are lesbians.** This myth was popularized by the book *Everything You Ever Wanted to Know About Sex but Were Afraid to Ask*. It is not true.

8. **Transvestites are homosexuals.** Most transvestites are, in fact, heterosexual, even though they enjoy dressing up as women.

9. **As you get older, the sex drive goes away.** The sex drive does decrease with age, but it does not stop. One of the biggest blocks for the elderly is that the men die before women do, and women are left without men to have sex with. Of women 65 to 74 years old, only 44 percent live with husbands. Widowhood increases very sharply after women turn 75, so sex is less available to these women, though perhaps not less desirable.

My advice is to keep two mistresses. Few men have the stamina for more.

—Ovid

———◆———

Male Sexual Myths

1. *The size of a flaccid penis indicates the size it will be when erect.* NOT true. You really can't tell from a flaccid penis what the beast will be like when it's awake. Even so, most men would be happier if their flaccid size were larger.

2. *The longer a man makes sex last, the more pleasure a woman gets.* Sometimes women like it shorter, too. One of the main reasons that women fake orgasms is to give the man permission to end an otherwise pleasurable sexual experience.

3. *A "real man" can get an instant hard-on anytime.* If this were true, then only 15-year-olds would be "real men." Response time slows as a man ages, and that's life.

4. *If a man turns down sex, there's something wrong with him.* This is one of the hardest myths for men to overcome. But sometimes a guy is just tired. Or satisfied. Let him have a night off, for goodness sakes!

5. *All men want is sex.* Men want to feel good about themselves, and sex often makes men feel that way. Thus, they often want sex. Okay, it's true—much of the time, men do want sex.

6. *The bigger a man's penis, the better.* Many women report feeling like their "cervix is being punched" by men who have extra-

long penises. Width seems more important to women than length, and of course, how good a lover a man is overall.

7. *Premature ejaculation is the result of being "weak-willed."* Sex therapists agree that "having more will power" is not the answer for increasing ejaculatory control. Sex therapist Bernie Zilbergeld says the problem is not a lack of will, but a lack of "focusing on their own sensations" and not knowing "what kind of adjustments [in the sexual activity] should be made."

8. *You really should be having exotic, "tantric" or other wildly varied sex.* Basically, this myth says that no matter how good your sex life is it should be better. Stop comparing your sex life to porn movies. Try to enjoy yourself.

The penis confers with human intelligence and has intelligence itself.

—Leonardo da Vinci

◆

What Women Want from Men

According to a 1995 poll, here's what women look for in men:

1. Eighty-eight percent look for men who are six feet tall or taller.

2. Eighty percent look for men with "imposing body massiveness."

3. Seventy-six percent look for a muscular, athletic build.

4. Seventy-two percent look for broad shoulders.

5. Sixty-five percent look for a large penis.

6. Sixty-four percent look for strong, muscular arms.

7. Sixty percent look for a small, tight rear.

8. Fifty-five percent look for a full head of hair.

9. Thirty-seven percent look for a sensual mouth.

10. Thirty-four percent look for narrow hips.

They also look for a square face, bushy eyebrows, a Roman nose, large eyes, narrow lips, and tan skin.

Love is blind.

—William Shakespeare

What Men Want from Women

A study from Auburn University about what men want from women should help drive female readers crazy. Men want:

1. Women who are sexually inexperienced, yet . . .

2. Women who really love sex.

3. Women who are slim and petite, yet . . .

4. Women who have really large breasts.

5. Women who are innocent, yet . . .

6. Women who are trustworthy and mature.

7. Women who are virtuous and reserved, yet . . .

8. Women who are flirtatious and adventuresome.

Best of luck!

> *A lady is one who never shows*
> *her underwear unintentionally.*
>
> —Lillian Day

———◆———

Who Rents Adult Videos?

In 1999 . . .

1. Men shopping alone accounted for 71 percent of adult-film rentals.

2. Men shopping with women accounted for 19 percent of adult-film rentals.

3. Men shopping with men accounted for 7 percent of adult-film rentals.

4. Women shopping with another woman accounted for 2 percent of adult-film rentals.

5. Women shopping alone accounted for less than 1 percent of adult-film rentals.

*The big difference between sex for money
and sex for free is that sex for money usually
costs a lot less.*

—Brendan Francis

---◆---

Lesbians Having Sex with Men

It would seem that sexual preferences exist on a continuum—you may be straight or gay, but how straight or gay are you? There seems to be a lot of middle ground, and the good folks at the Kinsey Institute have studied it—at least in lesbians.

1. Forty-four percent of lesbians have, at some point in their lives, labeled themselves heterosexual.

2. Fourteen percent of lesbians have, at some point in their lives, labeled themselves as bisexual.

3. Sixteen percent of lesbians have labeled themselves both heterosexual *and* bisexual at different points in their lives.

4. Twenty-six percent of lesbians have *always* labeled themselves as homosexual.

5. Seventy-four percent of women calling themselves lesbians have had sex with men.

6. Sixty-four percent of women calling themselves lesbians have had unprotected penile/vaginal intercourse.

7. Forty-two percent of women who have always called themselves lesbian have had sex with men.

8. Twenty-eight percent of women who have always called themselves lesbians have had unprotected penile-vaginal intercourse.

9. Two percent of women who have always called themselves lesbians have had unprotected penile-anal intercourse.

10. Fifteen percent of women who have always called themselves lesbians have had sex with behaviorally bisexual men (that is, guys who have sex with guys, whether they admit it or not).

Historically lesbians have lived not so much outside the law, both religious and secular, but beneath it.

—Jane Rul

—————◆—————

CHAPTER 9

Sex Play

Sex Games to Play with Your Partner

1. **Photo opportunities.** One of you is the photographer, the other the model, who must do what he or she is told and model in any position required (you can do this with or without film)!

2. **Blue movie star.** Put that video camera to work! Videotape your sexiest moves together and enjoy them together when you are done! If you are worried about the film showing up on some Web site, record over it once you've viewed it.

3. **Simon Says.** For a certain amount of time, whatever one partner says, *goes.* It's Simon Says with a sexual twist.

4. **Strip club at home.** Lower the lights, get into a sexy outfit, put on some throbbing music, and strip for your partner!

5. **The taste test.** Blindfold your partner and feed him or her bites of various foods, and see how he or she identifies them. Made popular by the film *9-1/2 Weeks*, when Mickey Rourke played this game with Kim Bassinger.

6. **The caress test.** Once again, blindfold your partner. Now caress his or her naked body with things you find around the house. How many of them can your partner identify?

7. **The gratification delay.** Have intercourse, but every time either of you get close to orgasm, stop and calm down, then start again. Do this for at least an hour, then let the orgasms rip!

8. **The stranger sex.** Go to a bar separately, and pretend to meet and seduce one another for the first time. See what opening lines work and which don't; seduce fully, and enjoy the rewards!

9. **The gender swap.** Men pretend to be women, and women pretend to be men. Take this as far as you desire before switching roles back to normal.

10. **The army of lovers.** Have your lover describe other lovers, real or imagined, and give them names, traits, favorite behaviors, and techniques. Then blindfold your lover and see if he or she can guess whom you are being.

11. **Variety hour.** Each of you writes down all the sex acts you've been curious about or secretly desired on little slips of paper and put them in a hat or bowl. Pull one out of the bowl, discuss it, and try it out if it is mutually agreeable. This can be a great way to share desires.

12. **Be still my . . . heart.** See how long you can be absolutely still while having intercourse.

13. **Pen pals.** Decide you will pretend to be strangers, and seduce each other in a steamy e-mail romance!

I used to be Snow White, but I drifted.

—Mae West

———◆———

Fetish Scene Lingo

BDSM. Bondage, discipline, and sadomasochism.

Lifestyle. People who consider BDSM a crucial part of their lives. For them, it is more than a "spice" in the bedroom.

Bottom. A person who is submissive during sexual play, but not in other circumstances outside sexual play.

Dom/dominant. A male who enjoys sexually dominating others.

Dominatrix. A female dominant; sometimes—though not always—a professional.

Domme. A female dominant.

D/S. Shorthand for Dominance and Submission. Any sex play that involves dominance and submission can be called D/S.

Female domination. A phrase used to describe when women are dominant.

Male domination. A phrase used to describe when men are dominant.

Master/Mistress. An honorific that submissives often use on their dominants, especially in established relationships.

Masochist. Someone who is sexually gratified by receiving pain.

Play. To "play" means to have a "scene" with another individual or individuals. The acting out of a shared fantasy.

S/M. Sadomasochism. Refers to sexual activities in which people experience sexual pleasure in the giving or receiving of pain.

Sadist. Someone who is sexually gratified by giving pain.

Safe word. A word, such as "safe," that would not normally be said during a scene. It means, "Stop, I really mean it." Having a safe word gives an "out" to any situation and keeps it safer.

Safe, sane, and consensual. The motto or creed of the BDSM community.

Scene. Used in two ways: "the scene," and "a scene." "The scene" is a subset of the fetish underworld. Someone might say, for instance, "New York has a great scene," meaning there are lots of fetish clubs and events. "A scene" is a fetish, fantasy-fulfillment interaction between two or more people. When you tie your submissive to a rack and whip him, it's "a scene."

Session. A single BDSM experience, or scene.

Slave. A submissive who is submissive to his or her dominant all the time.

Switch. A person who enjoys both dominating and submitting sexually, at different times.

Top. A dominant who controls the submissive during sexual play, but not in other circumstances outside sexual play.

Vanilla. Usually refers to conventional forms of sexual relations. Also refers to intimate interactions that do not include D/s or SM activity.

You can raise welts like nobody eltz.

—Tom Lehrer

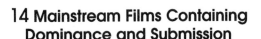

14 Mainstream Films Containing Dominance and Submission

One way to find out if your partner might enjoy playing with dominance and submission is to get one of these films that have D/s themes. You can find these in most video stores—one might be just the thing to perk up your next date!

1. **The Collector** (1965). Terrance Stamp, Samantha Eggar; director: William Wyler. A butterfly collector decides to expand his collection to include a woman.

2. **Belle de Jour** (1967). Catherine Deneuve, Jean Sorel, Michel Piccoli; director: Luis Buñuel. Catherine Deneuve plays a woman who can't bring herself to have sex with her husband, but who has a variety of kinky fantasies instead. Eventually, she becomes a prostitute while remaining chaste in her marriage.

3. **Last Tango in Paris** (1973). Marlon Brando, Maria Schneider; director: Bernardo Bertolucci. The classic. Good film, kinky sex.

4. **Maîtresse** (1976). Gérard Depardieu, Bulle Oier; director: Barbet Shroeder. Depardieu breaks into a professional dominatrix's apartment and falls in love with her.

5. **Liquid Sky** (1982) Anne Carlisle, Paula Sheppard; director: Slava Tsukerman. Weird and stylish, involving aliens who thrive on the chemicals people create during orgasm. Strange sex and dominance/submission.

6. **Videodrome** (1983) James Woods, Sonja Smits, Deborah Harr; director: David Cronenberg. A S/M relationship between the main characters.

7. **9-1/2 Weeks** (1986). Kim Bassinger, Mickey Rourke; director: Adrian Lyne. Kim Bassinger submits to Mickey Rourke in this erotic, popular film.

8. **Something Wild** (1986). Jeff Daniels, Melanie Griffith; director: Jonathan Demme. Fun with handcuffs.

9. ***Heart of Midnight*** (1988). Jennifer Jason Leigh; director: Matthew Chapman. Leigh inherits a building from her uncle that used to be a sex club, and starts remembering things . . .

10. ***Unforgiven*** (1992). Clint Eastwood, Gene Hackman, Morgan Freeman; director: Clint Eastwood. Has a flogging scene.

11. ***Whispers in the Dark*** (1992). Annabella Sciorra, Jamey Sheridan, Alan Alda; director: Christopher Crowe. A psychiatrist is working with a patient who has a submissive sexual relationship with her partner. Involves bondage.

12. ***Body of Evidence*** (1993). Madonna, Wilhem Dafoe, Joe Mantegna; director: Uli Edel. Madonna's famous movie of dominance and submission, Sadomasochism, and sex, including a hot-wax scene.

13. ***Exit to Eden*** (1994). Rosie O'Donnell, Dan Aykroyd; director: Garry Marshall. Not the best film ever made, takes place at an S/M vacation resort. Billed as a comedy but mostly just weird.

14. ***Bound*** (1996). Jennifer Tilly, Gina Gershon; directors: Andy Wachowski, Larry Wachowski. Tilly and Gershon have a hot lesbian relationship, with plenty of time in bondage, as they try to steal two million dollars from the Mob.

> *There is not a man who doesn't want to be a despot when he's excited.*
>
> —Marquis De Sade

Types of Condoms

- **Reservoir tip.** Most condoms have a nipple, or reservoir, at the tip to collect the ejaculate.

- **Blunt end.** These do not have a reservoir tip.

- **Lubricated.** Lubricated condoms are less likely to tear and can be easier to use. Some lubricated condoms also have nonoxynol-9, a spermicide, added to further help prevent pregnancy and to help stop the spread of sexually transmitted diseases. Spermicide has a bitter taste, however, so such condoms are usually not used for oral sex.

- **Unlubricated.** More likely to tear than lubricated condoms and do not have any spermicidal properties.

- **Lamb's skin.** These condoms are made of natural materials and are often said to conduct more sensation. They do *not* provide protection against the HIV virus. (Only latex condoms provide protection from HIV.)

- **Straight.** This type of condom doesn't follow the natural curves of the penis.

- **Shaped.** This condom is shaped more like a penis.

- **Colored.** Some people find that colored condoms spice up their sex life. Other people just find it strange to have a blaze-orange penis.

- **Large.** For those who need a bit larger size, several companies produce large-size condoms. Trojan makes one such condom, the Trojan-enz Large.

- **Extra large.** These condoms often need to be specially ordered, they are for especially well-endowed men. Trojan Magnum and MAXX are two such brands.

- **Narrow.** For narrower penises, these are less likely to slip or fall off.

- **Ultra-thin.** The biggest complaint men have about condoms is that they cut down on sensation, and ultra-thin condoms are designed to help avoid that. Ultra-thin condoms are quite thin (0.04–0.06 mm thick) and allow for increased transfer of heat and sensation.

- **Extra strong.** Good for people who do high-friction activities, such as anal sex, where a stronger condom is helpful.

- **Novelty condoms.** "French ticklers" and glow-in-the-dark condoms.

Withdrawal has an evil effect upon the woman's nervous condition.

—Margaret Sanger

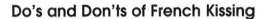

Do's and Don'ts of French Kissing

The term "French kiss" was first used in the 1920s, though, of course, tongue kissing has been around as long as there have been people and those people have had tongues. New couples may appreciate these tips, and couples who have been together for a long time may have forgotten about the simple pleasures of French kissing and may enjoy these reminders:

Do

- **Alternate being active and passive,** pushing your tongue into your partner's mouth and letting it into yours.

- **Explore different parts of your partner's mouth** with your tongue, and let your partner explore yours.

- **Touch your partner's face and lips** with your fingers while kissing—this adds a very erotic, intimate sensation for most people.

- **Relax your lips.** A relaxed lip is a soft lip! You can get your lips to relax by blowing a "raspberry." (Just don't do it in your partner's face.)

- **Breathe in unison.** If you can unobtrusively match your partner's breathing, breathing in when he or she does, and out when he or she does, you'll feel more connected and intimate during the kissing.

- **Experiment with having your eyes alternately open and closed,** so you can look at your partner, and then really focus on the sensation.

- **Make some sound.** Everybody likes to get positive feedback that their kissing is enjoyable. Your partner will appreciate your little moans and cries of pleasure.

- **Play with an ice-cube,** or a hard candy or mint. Such things can be fun to pass back and forth, or to run along each other's lips and tongue and teeth.

Don't

- **Don't be afraid to explore new sensations.** You may have forgotten about French kissing and experiencing new sensations, even French kissing a lover you've had for a long time. Let yourself enjoy the light-headedness, the tingles, or whatever sensations that might show up.

- **Don't burp.** This is critically important. If you have to burp, do whatever it takes not to gross your partner out. By all means, *never* burp directly into your partner's mouth.

- **By the same token, don't chew gum** or eat anything that gets gooey while French kissing.

- **Don't tighten up.** Tight lips aren't much fun to kiss, so don't press your lips together. Let go, and have fun!

Love begins with a smile, grows with a kiss, and ends with a teardrop.

—Anonymous

———◆———

10 Important Tantric Sex Positions

Studying Tantric sex, the ancient Indian meditative sexual practice, is a good way to make yourself feel bad about your sex life. No matter how hot your sex life is, these yogis are having a *much* better time than you, and it's spiritual, too! Tantric sex is prolonged sex, without a lot of movement—you get yourselves into the poses and savor the smallest of movements as the energy rises through the two of you. Together you enjoy each and every sensation. Men, here's a tip—as you near orgasm, prevent it by reaching your hand down between your legs, grasping your testicles, and pulling downward *gently*. Women, orgasm at will. But the idea for both sexes is to reach new heights of pleasure, not necessarily involving orgasm.

Like most exercise programs, you probably shouldn't fool around with some of these positions without first getting your doctor's permission. And you may need a good chiropractor to get out of them!

And another thing—when you read about Tantric sex, they'll almost always use the term *lingam* in place of "penis," and *yoni* in place of vagina. The woman may also be referred to as *kali*, or the *shakti*. The man may be referred to as *shiva*. *Asana* (pronounce "ah-sa-na") is Sanscrit for "pose." Knowing this will help you get through the basics, or at least be able to keep up during cocktail-party Tantric sex conversations.

1. **Hip rotation.** This isn't so much a seperate Tantric technique as it is a part of all Tantric techniques. After prolonged spiritual joining, you do hip rotation when you want to let your-

self finally orgasm. It's much the same for both sexes—tense the muscles of your butt, and move your hips in a "hula hoop" style rotating motion. This "corkscrewing" motion can be, um, highly stimulating.

2. **Kali Asana.** This is the basic "woman-on-top" position. The man lies on his back, and the woman mounts and rides him, sitting up on his body. This also exposes her clitoris for easy stimulation.

3. **Kukhapadma Asana.** The man sits on the floor or a cushion or some other supportive surface in the half-lotus position, or with his legs crossed if he's not quite spiritual enough to do a half-lotus. The woman mounts him and wraps her legs around his waist. They hold each other closely and touch tongues.

4. **Yoni Asana.** The man sits on a chair or couch with his knees bent and feet flat on the floor, and the woman mounts him, facing him, supporting them both by wrapping her arms around his torso. They look into each other's eyes, don't move much, and feel the energy build.

5. **Mounted Yantra Asana.** The woman lies on her back with her legs raised straight up in the air, more or less together, at a right angle to her body. The man sits facing her raised legs, straddling her body with his feet by the sides of her head, and enters her.

6. **Splitting Bamboo Asana.** In this pose the man enters the woman as in the Mounted Yantra Asana, but she puts on of her legs up by his head and lets the other one come down and drape over his upper thigh.

7. **Variegated Asana.** The man kneels and the woman squats before him, so he can enter her from behind. She wiggles in all directions as he rubs her body all over, starting with the palms of her hands.

8. **Mula Bandha Asana.** The man sits in full lotus position (you *can* sit in full lotus, can't you?) or simply has his legs crossed (loser). The woman mounts him, wrapping her legs around his hips, and he leans back supine, with her heels under his sacral area. They clasp each other by the wrists, then she leans back until she is supine as well. They gently pull themselves back up to the seated position, then back down to lying, over and over again until enlightenment and orgasm are reached. Piece of cake!

9. **Yab Yum Asana.** The man is in full lotus again, and the woman mounts him and wraps her legs around him. They stay upright this time, rocking toward ecstasy.

10. **Equal Peaks Asana.** The man sits upright, and the woman squats on him and inserts his lingam in her yoni, if you know what we mean. She then alternates straightening and bending her legs, one after another, back and forth, over and over.

When authorities warn you of the sinfulness of sex, there is an important lesson to be learned. Do not have sex with the authorities.

—Matt Groening

———◆———

The 9 Steps of the Taoist Thrusting Method for Men

The number nine is a very auspicious number in ancient Taoist (Chinese) texts about lovemaking, so you have to bring it into your sex life as well. The man thrusts in nine sets of ten thrusts each. It actually gets pretty intense, we are told.

1. Nine shallow thrusts, one deep thrust.

2. Eight shallow thrusts, two deep thrusts.

3. Seven shallow thrusts, three deep thrusts.

4. Six shallow thrusts, four deep thrusts.

5. Five shallow thrusts, five deep thrusts.

6. Four shallow thrusts, six deep thrusts.

7. Three shallow thrusts, seven deep thrusts.

8. Two shallow thrusts, eight deep thrusts.

9. One shallow thrust, nine deep thrusts.

Then start over, and repeat as many times as you can without ejaculating.

*Women complain about sex more than men.
Their gripes fall into two major categories:
(1) Not enough. (2) Too much.*

—Ann Landers

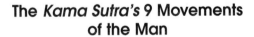

The *Kama Sutra's* 9 Movements
of the Man

1. **Moving forward.** That is, getting inserted properly.

2. **Churning.** The lingam is held in the hand and moved all around in the yoni.

3. **Piercing.** When most of the thrusting attention is to the upper part of the vagina.

4. **Rubbing.** When most of the thrusting attention is to the lower part of the vagina.

5. **Pressing.** A "press-and-hold" posture of the lingam in the yoni.

6. **Giving a blow.** Almost full or full withdrawal, then a sudden hard thrust.

7. **Blow of the boar.** When only part of the vagina is stimulated by the penis.

8. **Blow of the bull.** When both sides of the vagina are rubbed.

9. **Sporting of a sparrow.** Lots of thrusting, right near the end of intercourse.

Men are those creatures with two legs
and eight hands.

—Jayne Mansfield

———◆———

Tantric Sex Workshops

If you must know more about Tantric sex, there are plenty of people happy to teach you. Some resources for the curious include:

- *Tantra.com:* 800-9-TANTRA; http://www.tantra.com
- *Muirs' Source School of Tantra:* (808) 572-8364; http://www.sourcetantra.com/

- *Oceanic Tantra with Kutira and Raphael:* (808) 572-6006; http://www.oceanictantra.com/

- *Celebrations of Love:* (415) 924-5483; http://www.celebrationsoflove.com/

- *Margot Anand's SkyDancing:* (415) 381-0844; http://www.skydancing.com/

- *Tantrika International:* (888) TANTRIKA; http://www.tantrika.com

- *New York Open Center:* (212) 219-2527; http://www.opencenter.org/

- *Richard and Diana Daffner:* (808) 244-4103; http://www.TantraTaiChi.com

- *School of Tantra:* http://www.schooloftantra.com

*For some, sex leads to sainthood; for others
it is the road to hell . . . all depends
on one's point of view.*

—Henry Miller

---◆---

7 Types of Kissing
from the *Kama Sutra*

Vatsyayana, the author of the *Kama Sutra*, didn't limit his writing to intercourse—he also talked about kissing. Here are some kisses from the *Kama Sutra* that you can include in your sex play:

1. **The bent kiss.** Lovers bend their heads toward each other while they kiss.

2. **The straight kiss.** Both partners bring their lips in direct and full contact with the other.

3. **The pressed kiss.** The lower lip is pressed hard into the partner's lips.

4. **The turned kiss.** One partner turns the head of the other for the kiss.

5. **The clasping kiss.** One partner takes both lips of the other between his or her own.

6. **Fighting of the tongue.** French kissing, *Kama Sutra* style.

7. **Other.** The *Kama Sutra* recommends kissing "the forehead, the eyes, the cheeks, the throat, the bosom, the breasts, the lips and the interior of the mouth." Kiss other places at your own risk.

. . . To this we would add the "olfactory kiss," where the lovers touch noses while kissing and enjoy the sensation and each other's scents.

> *Two people kissing always look like fish.*
>
> —Andy Warhol

Body Piercings for Men

There's more than one way to pierce a penis, as it turns out. Here's a lexicon of piercings for men:

1. **Nipple piercings.** Legend has it that nipple piercings go back at least as far as Roman times, when centurions would have

nipple piercings as signs of their bravery and as anchors for their capes (ouch!).

2. **The Prince Albert piercing.** Another brilliant Victorian invention, the Prince Albert piercing is named after Prince Albert, who is said to have had one. The piercing enters near the head and out the opening at the front of the penis. A ring is then inserted. Apparently Prince Albert and other Victorian men wore such a piercing so they could use it as an anchor to hold their penises properly in place and flat in the tight pants of the time. Oh yeah, it's also apparently quite pleasurable for the man and his partner during sex.

3. **The dydoe.** These piercings are said to return some of the sensation lost through circumcision. A small bar with balls or studs on each end is pierced through the upper edge of the glans, front to back, near the shaft of the penis.

4. **The ampallang.** This piercing is indiginous to the areas surrounding the Indian Ocean. The piercing is done through the center of the head of the penis, horizontally, above the urethra. Rings or studs may be attached to this bar, to aid stimulation during sex. This piercing was often done ritually as part of a puberty rite.

5. **The apadravya (also known as apadavra).** This piercing is a bar placed through the head of the penis vertically or just behind the head, top to bottom. Said to be very stimulating to the ladies.

6. **Piercing the frenum.** The frenum is the loose piece of skin just behind and below the head of the penis. This piercing can be made either stimulating or chastity enforcing. A ring through the frenum is stimulating and can be flipped up over the head of the penis both to stimulate the woman or to be worn as a penis ring. If the frenum ring has a lock or other

large item put through it, intercourse is impossible. If it is attached to another piercing at the base of the penis, even erection is impossible.

7. **The hafada.** The hafada piercing is an ancient Arab custom done at puberty in the belief that it would prevent the testicles from rising into the body. It is a piercing of the side of the scrotum.

8. **The guiche.** This is a piercing behind the testicles, between the testicles and the anus. It is said to intensify pleasure if gently pulled on during orgasm.

9. **The ears.** Yes, you can still pierce your ears. But it might seem kind of boring.

I think men who have a pierced ear are better prepared for marriage. They've experienced pain and bought jewelry.

—Rita Rudner

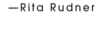

Body Piercings for Women

1. **Nipple piercings.** Victorian women often had nipple piercings, strange as it may seem. They had rings to increase the size of their nipples and to make them more prominent.

2. **Navel piercings.** A pierced navel was a sign of royalty among ancient Egyptians. Today it is available to anyone who wants it, royalty or not. This piercing has no direct sexual conse-

quences—it doesn't increase sexual stimulation in any way. The piercing is of the fold of skin above the navel and it takes approximately six weeks to heal.

3. **The clitoral hood.** The clitoral hood (the equivalent of the male foreskin) is a common place for vaginal piercings. Note that this is *not* the same as having the clitoris pierced (see number 4). Often a ring is put through this piercing with a small ball that rests on and stimulates the clitoris.

4. **The clitoris piercing.** Most people who know a little about piercing think of this when they think of genital piercing of women, but they usually are confusing this piercing with that of the clitoral hood. Clitoral piercings are much rarer, as they are quite painful and there is the possibility of nerve damage and loss of sensation.

5. **Labia piercings.** The piercing of the outer labia with bars or rings is mostly decorative, though some women do hang light weights from them for stimulation.

6. **Facial piercings.** Though not technically "body" piercings, and actually for both women and men, facial piercings make a statement to everyone you meet. Some have said such piercings are best for those who are reconciled to diminished employment opportunities, or those who work in high-tech start-ups. The nose, the area above and below the lips, and the eyebrows can be pierced.

7. **The tongue.**

8. **The ears.**

Always have piercings done by a qualified professional.

If a woman seeks education it is probably because her sexual apparatus is malfunctioning.

—Friedrich Nietzsche

———◆———

The Most Common Sexual Fantasies— and Just How Common They Are

An extensive study at UCLA found a lot of useful information about sexual fantasies that you need to know. Some of these statistics won't surprise you, but some probably will.

1. Not surprisingly, approximately an equal number—98.1 percent of men and 97.2 percent of women—said they fantasized about touching and kissing sensuously.

2. Interestingly, more men than women fantasized about being seduced—87 percent of men and 80.2 percent of women fantasized about being seduced.

3. In a reversal of what we might expect in a world where much older men routinely date and marry much younger women, more men than women fantasized about a much older partner—57.4 percent of men vs. 36.8 percent of women.

4. More than half (55.6 percent) of men fantasized about anal intercourse, while less than half that number (25.5 percent) of women did so.

5. The same percentage of men fantasized about being involved in an orgy, while less than half that number (29.2 percent) of women admitted to doing so.

6. In the realm of dominance and submission, 44.4 percent of men fantasized about being forced to submit, while 36.2 percent of women did so.

7. Meanwhile, 42.6 percent of men fantasized about forcing a partner to submit, while roughly half that number, 22.6 percent of women fantasized about the same thing.

8. And some bad news for men and mate-swapping: While 25.9 percent of men fantasized about mate-swapping, less than half that number (11.3 percent) of women did.

9. Although 46.2 percent of women fantasized about being rescued from danger by one who would become a lover, only 25 percent of men admitted to doing so.

10. On to the world of sadomasochism—22.2 percent of men admitted to fantasizing about whipping or beating a partner. Less than a fifth that number, 3.8 percent, of women did so.

11. And 18.5 percent of men fantasized about being whipped or beaten by a sexual partner; 4.7 percent of women had those same fantasies.

12. The same percentage (18.5) of men fantasized about being sexually degraded; less than half that number, 7.5 percent, of women fantasized about being sexually degraded.

13. Meanwhile, 9.3 percent of men fantasized about degrading a sexual partner, while less than a third of that number of women (3 percent) did so. So, there are 3 percent of women to fulfill 18.5 percent of men's fantasies to be sexually degraded. Those ain't good odds.

14. And 13 percent of men fantasized about being tortured by a sex partner, while only 4.7 percent of women did so.

15. Meanwhile, 9.3 percent of men fantasized about torturing a sex partner, while less than a fourth that number of women

(1.9 percent) did so. There's 1.9 percent of women to fulfill 13 percent of men's sex fantasies about being tortured. No wonder professional dominatrixes are always in demand!

16. And on to bisexuality: 33 percent of women admitted to having homosexual fantasies if heterosexual, or heterosexual fantasies if homosexual. Only 18.9 percent of men admitted to the same thing. That's good news for men trying to find a woman who might be interested in an erotic three-way with one of her female friends—your chances of finding a woman who at least fantasizes about it is one in three!

17. Not one man in the study admitted to fantasizing about having sexual relations with animals; 2.8 percent of women did. Now that's *really* sick.

My breasts are beautiful, and I gotta tell you, they've gotten a lot of attention for what is a relatively short screen time.

—Jamie Lee Curtis

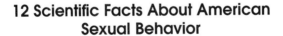

12 Scientific Facts About American Sexual Behavior

A University of Chicago study of over 3,500 Americans ages 18 to 59 released in 1994 found out some facts about Americans that are considered to be more accurate than any other study.

1. Fifty-four percent of men think about sex daily; 19 percent of women do.

2. Eighty-three percent of Americans have zero or only one sexual partner a year.

3. The average man has a six sexual partners over his lifetime.

4. The average woman has two sexual partners over her lifetime.

5. Approximately one third of Americans have sex twice a week or more.

6. Approximately one third of Americans have sex a few times a month.

7. Approximately one third of Americans have sex a few times a year, or not at all.

8. Almost 40 percent of married people say they have sex twice a week.

9. Twenty-five percent of single people say they have sex twice a week.

10. Seventy-five percent of married men say they have never cheated on their spouse.

11. Eighty-five percent of married women say they have never cheated on their spouse.

12. Three percent of adult Americans have never had sex.

*I know nothing about sex, because
I was always married.*

—Zsa Zsa Gabor

Notable Porn Directors

1. **Robert Black.** Controversial by some people's assessment, "twisted" by others, and "wacky" by his own, Robert Black is a young producer who is making it bigger all the time. He goes for the strange—one film has a black-faced pimp with a white penis, an infantilism scene, and an electrocution scene. Not for the faint of heart. Some of his films: *Abuse of Power, Cellar Dwellers, Fuck My Dirty Shit Hole: The Movie, Moral Degeneration.*

2. **Andrew Blake.** A painter, director, and photographer before becoming a porn director, his artistic sensibilities fill every film. He says his priorities in film are "women, sex, fashion and architecture—in that order." The sex is beautiful and artistic, yet still explicit and erotic. His work is often recommended for couples, but some women are put off by the preponderance of female-female sex (most men aren't). He's sometimes called the Helmut Newton of porn films. Some of his films: *Les Femmes Erotique, Hidden Obsessions, Night Trips (1 and 2), Paris Chic (1 and 2), Possessions.*

3. **Ernest Greene.** With his well-thought-out and brilliantly produced fetish and S/M films, Ernest Green obviously cares about what he is doing. There's no sexual intercourse (it's faked, when it's there at all) for legal reasons. Some of his films: *Contract for Service, Lydia's Web, Bondage of the Rising Sun, Plaything (1 and 2), Where the Boys Aren't.*

4. **Veronica Hart.** A porn-actress turned director, Hart also brings female sensibilities to the often formulaic world of sex films. Some of her films: *Adam and Eve's House Party (1 and 2), Fountain of Innocence, Lady Luck, The Wrong Snatch.*

5. **John Leslie.** Leslie is known for his great camerawork and tight editing. His work is explicit, his stories good, and his soundtracks excellent. Some of his films: *Curse of the Catwoman, Anything that Moves, Chameleons, Fresh Meat: A Ghost Story.*

6. **Michael Ninn.** His work is described as "moody" and "atmospheric" as well as "awesome" and "unbelievable"; like a glossy magazine (but with explicit sex). His movies even use computerized special effects! In an interview he says, "Just don't call me an esoteric Carl Jung fanatic." The images in his films might make you think he is. Some of his films: *Latex, Sex, Sex 2, Shock, Fade to Blue, Diva (1–3).*

7. **Candida Royalle.** A former sex-film actress herself, Royalle's films emphasize real sex, real female orgasms, and real female pleasure. For those who are tired of fake-looking women having fake-looking orgasms in porn, or orgasming from things that would never arouse a "real-world" woman, her films are for you. Some of her films: *The Bridal Shower, My Surrender, One Size Fits All.*

8. **Michael Zen.** Strong stories and well-made films. Great if you want some story with your sex. Some of his films: *Blue Movie, Censored, Cinesex (1 and 2), Expose Me Again.*

> *Pornography is the attempt to insult sex, to do dirt on it.*
>
> —D. H. Lawrence

The Best Opening Lines of All Time

As the authors of *How to Succeed with Women* and *How to Succeed with Men*, we often get asked "What is the best opening line?" Here it is:

"Hi." According to a University of Chicago study, this is the best opening line there is, followed by "How do you like the band?" (but only if a band is, in fact, playing). All the cutesie lines you've heard—"Can I borrow your cell phone? I want to call heaven and tell them I found the missing angel"—don't work any better and usually work quite a bit worse. Even if the cutesie line does work, you are still left with the same basic problem—here's a human being in front of me, what do I say? "Hi" works best at getting you to that point. After that, you need to know how to flirt. See the next list!

10 Essential Flirting Moves You Must Know

1. **Smiling.** You must smile. You probably think you smile now, but you don't, really. You should practice your smile in the mirror—to be big enough to be noticed, your smile will probably have to be bigger than you are used to.

2. **Getting caught looking.** Most people look away when the object of their desire looks at them. If you want to let that person know you are interested, when he or she catches you looking, smile, hold eye contact a moment longer, then look away.

3. **Waving.** A little wave to someone who caught you looking, along with a smile, is a nonintrusive, very flirty way to say "hello."

4. **Winking.** You can wink at someone from across the room, or wink at someone during a conversation. If he or she says something funny, or someone else does something silly, you can give a wink as a way of sharing a little moment for just the two of you, as if the two of you are in on some private joke no one else is aware of.

5. **Asking "What's the story behind that?"** You can ask the question about any special or unusual thing your quarry is wearing or carrying. Examples: "That's really a neat bracelet you are wearing. What's the story behind that?" or "That's a really great briefcase. What's the story behind that?" Even if there isn't much of one, it's given you some conversation.

6. **Holding eye contact.** While you are conversing with your new friend, you want to be sure to have eye contact at least some of the time. At least once it's a good idea to hold the eye contact a little "too long," just a fraction too long, so there's a brief, more intimate moment between you.

7. **Nonintrusive touching.** This can be as simple as placing your hand lightly on his or her hand for a moment, or touching his or her back for a moment as you walk to a table to sit down. Just do this a couple of times on the first flirting interaction—if the person pulls away, don't do it again.

8. **Checking him/her out.** Checking out someone's body must be done properly, especially if you are checking out a woman. The goal is for your new friend to feel complimented that you noticed his or her body, not objectified like some piece of meat.

   You do this by making eye contact, then quickly, in less than a second, passing your eyes down and then up over his or her body, then back to looking in the eyes. It should happen quickly, and you should be unashamed of taking a glance. Just don't do it too often.

9. **Using the "good-bye compliment."** If you are shy, flirting with the "good-bye compliment" may be just the thing you need. On your way out, you simply go up to the person you want to flirt with and say something like, "Hi, I have to go now, but before I did, I really wanted to let you know that you have a really great sense of style and that I noticed it. I wish I had more time to spend with you, but I have to go." Then leave. This allows you to build your confidence in approaching people, without having to take the risk of rejection—after all, you have to leave, you couldn't stay even if they wanted you to! (Some people also ask for phone numbers at this point.)

10. **Stopping while it's still fun.** Remember, flirting should be fun, and you should leave the flirting interaction feeling victorious. Most people leave their flirting interactions feeling like failures because they don't stop until it stops being fun. If you stop flirting on a high point, while it's still fun, your new friend will feel good when thinking of you and will want to see you again.

I hate the whole sex scene. I put a bottle over the head of anybody who tries to chat me up.

—Toyah Wilcox

Best Places to Meet a Mate

Most people want to know where to meet a mate. The best places to meet people are places that you go to on a regular basis at a regular time, such as the coffee shop you go to every morning, the bookstore/cafe you go to every Thursday evening, or the gym you go to every Monday, Wednesday, and Friday afternoons. When you become a regular, you get to know the staff and the other regulars, some of whom will be possible dating partners.

Aside from routine places, we suggest you check out

1. Art openings

2. Fundraising parties and events

3. Art fairs

4. Wine-tasting parties

5. Film festivals

6. Singles parties

7. Church and church events

8. Museum singles nights

9. Yoga classes

10. Coed sports leagues

11. Roller blading

12. Martial-art courses

13. The singles volunteer network

14. Volunteering for political campaigns

15. Volunteering for nonprofit community organizations (for example, hospitals or publicly funded radio stations)

16. Nature walks

17. Bird-identification classes

18. Alternative-health classes

19. Toastmasters

20. Acting classes

21. The Society for Creative Anachronisms

22. Renaissance fairs

23. Psychic fairs

24. Personal-growth seminars (for example: Shadow Work Seminars, the Forum, MORE University, Miracle of Love)

25. New Age spiritual communities

26. Meditation classes

27. Support groups for any addiction or health problem

28. Having friends set you up with their exes, relatives, co-workers, friends, etc.

29. Adventure travel groups

30. Cigar nights

31. Book-discussion groups

32. Waiting in a line

33. MENSA meetings

34. Film-discussion groups

35. Book clubs and salons

*Once a boy becomes a man, he's a man
all his life, but a woman is only sexy until
she becomes your wife.*

—Al Bundy

The Top 10 Love Potions

Kids, don't try these at home.

1. Mandrake

The most popular of the historical plants used in love potions throughout time is mandrake. It has been noted in folklore from the Assyrians, Babylonians, Egyptians, Romans, and Chinese as an important part of love potions. The Greeks associated mandrake with Aphrodite, the goddess of love, and often referred to her as "Mandragoris." Mandrake has been used both as an aphrodisiac and as an element that helps someone to attract a lover.

2. Animal Testicles

Many primitive societies, such as the Australian aborigines, use kangaroo testicles in love potions. Other traditions use beaver testicles. Other animal parts have also been used. During the Medieval period, young women would use bats' blood to attract a man.

3. Human Body Products

Many rituals to attract love include using semen, menstrual blood, and excrement. Let's not discuss them.

4. Herbs

Love-herb combinations are created by mixing herb mixtures with wax and then burning the wax in a ceremonial manner.

5. Love Candles

Candles are a ritual instrument often used in witchcraft rituals to invoke spirits. When powdered vervain and passion flower are added to a red candle, it is said to be able to invoke love.

6. Passion Candle

Add myrtle and cloves to a red candle. This is said to invoke passion in relationships.

7. Marriage Candle

Add orange blossoms, orris root, and anise seed to a red candle. This is said to assist in strengthening an existing relationship or to help attract a lover who will propose.

8. Love Incense

Along with candles, incense is often used in rituals as a way to invoke spirits. Many types can be burned to invoke energies or spirits. Here is one receipe:

- 1 oz. rose petals

- 1/4 oz. sweet bugle

- 1/2 oz. cinnamon

- 1/4 oz. anise seed

- 1/4 oz. frankincense

- 1 oz. powdered sandlewood

- 1/4 tsp. saltpeter

- 2 drams benzoin

9. Love Oil

Many people involved in witchcraft use different combinations of herbs and oils as a way to invoke spiritual powers. After creating a love oil potion it is recommended that the seeker place the oil on the forehead and on the navel. It is also suggested that love oil be used when bathing.

- Mix equal parts of loverage herb and grated lemon peel, from fresh lemons.

- Add 2 tablespoons of the herb and lemon mixture with 2 ounces of olive oil.

- Add a small piece of lodestone to each bottle of love oil made.

10. Attraction Oil

This potion is to be used on the forehead, genitals, and heart to attract a lover of your dreams

- Mix 2 tablespoons of red rose, lavender, and jasmine together.

- Add 2 ounces of olive oil.

- Add a small piece of orris root to each bottle made.

Keep your eyes half open before marriage and half shut afterwards.

—Benjamin Franklin

8 Ways for Women to Flirt with Their Feet

Some men have a foot fetish. Many body-language experts claim that the feet convey sexual signals. If you want to grab the attention of a man you need to be prepared. Here are several ways to have your feet do the talking.

1. **Play footsie with the guy.** Caress a man's foot under a table while pretending to be innocent. You can rest your foot against his or rub it. He will be shocked and you'll hope he'll respond in kind.

2. **While standing, bend over and adjust your heels** or stockings, touching your feet in a seductive manner while displaying your legs.

3. **Heels, heels, heels.** Wear high heels; it drives men crazy. One caveat: do not wear heels that make you taller than your date.

4. **Get a pedicure today.** Beautiful feet are often considered sexy.

5. **While sitting on the couch,** wrap your feet around his neck and pull him toward you.

6. **While sitting in a restaurant,** place your foot in his crotch and rub gently. If he doesn't respond to this erotic ploy then he must be dead.

7. **Dangle the sex.** As you sit with your legs crossed dangle one heel, thus exposing the underside of your foot. Look deep into the man's eyes as you do so.

8. **Practice your yoga.** If you practice yoga long enough you will be able to place your foot in the back of your head, thus looking like a true-blue contortionist. Another impressive move is to place your foot in your mouth (literally).

There is no greater nor keener pleasure than that
of bodily love—and none which is more irrational.

—Plato

Scams Men Pull to Meet
and Date Women

Over the past five years we have been teaching men of all ages and
all backgrounds how they can succeed with women. During that time
we've heard dozens of bizarre scams and ploys men have used when
trying to meet and bed women. We have included several for your
amusement. Women should read this list as a way to understand the
desperate measures men will go to meet you and date you and get
you in bed. Women can also use this list as a way to protect themselves
from being manipulated by the packs of horny jerks out there.

1. The Lost-Dog Ploy

One man would go to his local dog park and pretend to have
lost his dog. He often found sympathetic women who would help
him search for his dog and offer hugs to support his emotionally
upset state. He claims that several women offered him their phone
numbers to help ease his pain.

2. The Dead-Friend Ploy

Another man we know pretended to be grief stricken, claiming that his best friend had recently died. This is even more immoral
than the previous scam. The man claimed that it worked every time.

3. Conducting a Survey

Several students in the Los Angeles area banded together
and decided to run a fake survey on women. Armed with clip-

boards and survey questions they went out on a Friday morning around 1:00 A.M. and asked the most beautiful women to take a few moments to fill out a survey. But what did they ask? Sexual questions, of course. They then used the answers to attempt to seduce the women. This is not ethical and has no academic bearing, but they had fun in the process.

4. Teaching a Class to Get Some Ass

We've also known men who became instructors at university and workshop levels with the sole purpose of meeting women. One man taught an extension course at his local community college on auto mechanics and ended up dating a woman from the class. Another man offered to tutor students in chemistry, but would work only with female students. This scam has been used by many men to meet women.

5. Palm Reading

Many men look for a scam in which they can extract personal information about a woman and then use the information to seduce her. This pattern of behavior is the common thread among many of the scams listed. We've heard from our male students that women interested in the New Age are often gullible. As a result some men have taken up an interest in New Age things as a way to meet women. A few of the "get-laid" books available mention learning palm reading as a way to seduce women. They claim that by touching a woman's hand and being able to "predict" her future, they can use the experience as a romantic interaction that can lead to the woman falling starry-eyed for the male palm reader. This method has not been proven to work.

6. The Photographer Hoax

The classic scam is for a man to pretend to be a photographer and approach a woman he finds attractive on the beach and ask for her phone number so he can set up a photo shoot. This scam is as old as the hills, and it is hard to believe that it works. Still, several men claim that this scam works for them. They approach women by pointing their camera at them, even if they do not have film in the camera. They claim to be a talent scout or to work for a modeling agency and often offer to photograph the woman for free. When the woman arrives for the photo session the "photographer" uses the time as a seduction opportunity. Advice to women: Stay clear of men trying to photograph you.

7. The Band-Member Hoax

We all know that women are attracted to musicians. This is an inarguable fact. Along with the photographer scam, many men have attempted to pretend they are with a band. They approach a woman and lie about who they really are in an attempt to impress a woman gullible enough to think that a band member is really interested. From there, the man usually tries to manipulate a woman into undressing or into having sex right then and there. Smart women should look for ways in which a man can prove his credibility before even considering falling for this ploy.

8. The Relative-of-Someone-Famous Hoax

Along with being part of a famous band, some men also lie that they are related to someone famous as a way to impress a woman. This scam is much harder to prove, as a man does not have to look even remotely like the celebrity to be related to him or her. This scam has been done for decades to impress gullible women into believing that if they sleep with the relative of someone famous perhaps it will lead to meeting the famous person. However, most women end up crushed when they realize the whole thing was a lie and was done only to manipulate them into bed.

9. The Foreign-Accent Hoax

We knew one man who pretended he was from a foreign country as a way to appear more interesting to women. He was in college and used this ploy to stand out from the other guys at his university. This scam worked for him, and he met and dated several women.

However, the whole thing backfired when he started to become interested in a woman and he had a difficult time keeping his "accent" consistent. The woman eventually found out that he had lied and broke up with him. This scam is not recommended.

> *It's not money, it's not politics—it's who controls*
> *the pussy that controls the world.*
>
> —Larry Flynt

Top 12 Sexy Outfits for Men and Women

For those erotically challenged individuals reading this, style always makes the man or woman. The mind, however, can be a terribly dark and twisted place, as can be the demented realm of sexual fantasy. It is with respect for the inner hell that the following list was created.

Women

1. Dress as a **horse-racing jockey**, along with black protective helmet, boots, and riding crop. The man dresses as a horse, along with saddle, reins, and bit in mouth.

2. A **Victorian mistress** with corset, six-inch spiked heels, garter belt and thigh high stockings, silk gloves, lace, dark lips, pale skin, and a whip.

3. **Sexy nurse**, **naughty doctor**, or **sexy French maid**.

4. **Classic stern teacher** with glasses, pink polyester suit, ruler, black bra, and black panty hose.

5. **Hula girl**, with grass skirt, coconuts as a bra, dancing bare-foot. Or dress as a **belly dancer** with chain belt, and an *I Dream of Jeanie* costume.

6. **Latex, latex, latex**: PVC, short skirts, two-piece bathing suits, halter tops, leather pants, cat suits, bare midriff tops, and knee-high boots.

Men

1. **Construction worker** with blaze orange safety vest, tool belt, safety helmet, and steel-toed boots.

2. **Cock ring with leather anal harness,** temporary tattoos covering legs and chest, and a demon mask.

3. **Macho cowboy** with leather chaps, holster with squirt gun, cowboy hat, boots, and fringe vest.

4. **Business mogul** with classic Armani power suit and tie.

5. **Macho athlete** with lycra riding shorts and no shirt, exposing a six-pack stomach and burly physique. Option two is a **race car driver** getup.

6. **A man in uniform** (policemen, fireman, drill sergeant, plumber, Boy Scout, or sailor).

I know right away when it's lust. I mean, guys know. It's immediate. It's purely physical.

—Jason Priestly

The 4 Types of Swinging

Swinging is a complex art. There are many types of swingers and many rules that should be followed when participating in a swinging session. There are more than five million swingers in the United States. If you plan to get into swinging you'd better understand the different styles so you don't offend someone or push too hard or too fast without permission.

1. Open Swinging

This type of swinging is when several couples swap partners and have sex in the same room. This allows for the male and female partners to watch their partners make love to a different person, which some find to be a turn-on. This type of swinging is popular when bisexual women make love as the husbands enjoy watching.

2. Soft Swinging

With the rise in HIV, many swingers have ceased having sexual intercourse with anyone other than their committed partner. Soft swinging does not involve sexual intercourse. It can include sexual activities such as mutual masturbation, oral sex, watching, and being watched.

3. Group Swinging

Group swinging is the closest thing to an orgy that is done in swing communities. In these situations four or more couples swap partners and have sex in one or two rooms. Those interested in voyeurism and exhibitionism tend to enjoy this form of swinging. It is different than open swinging in that it is much more intense, sexual intercourse happens, and couples are often placed in separate rooms.

4. Closed Swinging

Closed swinging is the most relaxed form of swinging. In these situations two couples swing in separate rooms. This lends privacy to individuals so that they can feel more relaxed and uninhibited.

Bigamy is having one wife too many.
Monogamy is the same.

—Anonymous, but quoted by Erica Jong

———◆———

6 Love Spells

1. To Attract Office Romance

Take a piece of yellow chalk and draw a pentagram in each drawer of your desk. While drawing the pentagram chant out loud, "Power and influence come to me, let (the person you are trying to attract) be in love with me." Do this daily.

2. For a Lover Who Is Oversexed

Here is a spell to calm down your oversexed lover: Place a gardenia in your lover's champagne. Next, chant to yourself, "Flower of love, cool the lust and calm the passion."

3. To Get a Lover to Commit

Take a mirror that your lover has looked into. Break the mirror into pieces before looking into it. Next, bury the broken pieces with a plant in your backyard or in a flower pot. And then each Friday evening water the plant with tea water made from spikenard herb. While watering the plant repeat the name of your potential lover over and over.

4. The Witchcraft Holding Rite

This ritual is done to get someone to stay in a relationship. It should be done only if you love the person greatly and want him/her to be with you permanently.

- Find a way to secure a fingernail or toenail clipping and a few strands of hair from the person.

- Save the nail cutting in a small bottle with a stopper.

- Place nine sharp sewing needles in the bottle as well.

- Urinate in the bottle and then hold the bottle in your left hand while repeating the person's name six times.

- Repeat this ritual weekly until the relationship is settled.

- If you want to break off the relationship, smash the bottle against a tree.

5. When You Are Not Attracted to Your Lover

Purchase a fully blooming rose. Place the rose on an altar and then begin chanting, "Forever lovers (mention your name and your lover's name) with each other forever." Next, scatter the rose petals in your bed and sleep with your lover on top of the rose petals for three consecutive nights. At midnight on the third night, take all of the petals and place them under your lover's pillow. Keep them under the pillow for three more nights.

6. To Get a Lover to Propose

Take your lover to church on a Sunday. When he/she is deep in prayer take a thread from his/her clothing. While at church, hold the thread in your right hand and chant to yourself, "Marry me on this spot, or love won't linger with this knot."

7. To Attract a Man

Here is a traditional spell to attract a man. An unmarried woman takes the bladebone of a shoulder of a lamb. She must take a knife and stick the knife through the bone once per night for nine nights. Each night after the knife ritual, she is to say out loud, "Tis not the bone I mean to stick, but my lover's heart I meant to prick. Wishing him neither rest nor sleep, til he come to me to speak."

For a woman to be loved, she usually ought to be naked

—Pierre Cardin

The 9 Step Marriage Ritual

This ritual is complicated, but many claim that it is highly effective. For maximum benefits, it is recommended that this ritual be done on a Friday night when the moon is in its waxing phase.

You first need to assemble several materials to complete this ritual.

- Red ribbon, 21 inches
- Incense that invokes sensuality
- White linen, 19-inch piece
- Mixture of one part orange blossoms and one part mandrake
- Two cloth dolls, which represent to you the potential groom and bride
- Seven red candles

Step 1: The ritual begins by lighting three red candles. This is done with eyes shut and while the incense is burning.

Step 2: Tie the hands of each doll to the opposite hand of the other doll using the red ribbon, thus connecting the dolls representing the bride and the groom. The remaining ribbon is to be tied around the waists of the dolls. As you use the red ribbon chant:

> The bride and groom, now marriage can come true
> In both hearts and minds it will be true (state bride's name and then groom's name) This couple shall marry.

Then lay the dolls between the three lit candles.

Step 3: Light the remaining four red candles and say:

> As I light these candles the bride and groom become one
> (State bride and groom's name). They shall now marry forever.

Step 4: Sprinkle the mandrake and orange-blossom mixture over the dolls. While doing so say:

> This couple shall become one, I will this wedding to be
> The fate between the two of you is sealed
> Your wedding day is upon us.

Step 5: Allow the candles to burn for six minutes. During this time imagine the couple exchanging wedding vows and imagine the actual wedding taking place in as vivid detail as possible.

Step 6: Do this entire ritual three times per week for four weeks. On the last day of the ritual wrap the dolls up in linen and hide them until the day of the actual wedding.

*Marriage still remained the most holy
of institutions in America; even the rising rate
of divorce seemed chiefly to be for the purpose
of remarriage.*

—Andrew Sinclair, *The Better Half* (1965)

The Dumbest Pickup Lines of All Time*

Pickup lines are a dreaded art form. They are like the Jerry Springer Show. You don't want to watch, but can't quite resist, even though it is unbelievably dumb and predictable. At their very best pickup lines are amusing. At their worst they can be offensive and get a guy slapped. They are an important part of our cultural dating mythology and any true-blue sex lover must have an understanding of some of the dumbest and cheesiest lines to use at parties, on friends, and on men and women they meet.

1. Hi, I may not be Fred Flintstone, but I'd certainly like to make your bed rock.

2. Would you believe me if I told you I'm an angel, and God sent me down here on a special mission just to give you a kiss?

3. Let's do breakfast tomorrow. Should I call you or nudge you?

4. If I could rewrite the alphabet, I would put you between *f* and *ck*.

---

*A note to men: Louis and Copeland will not be held responsible if you are actually dumb enough to try these lines on women at a bar or anywhere else. We are released of all legal responsibility for any lack of sex that might follow.

274

5. You look yummy. You must bring new meaning to the word "edible."

6. Nice shoes, do you want to fuck?

7. I've heard that sex is a killer. Do you want to die happy?

8. I would like you to attend my party, and then we can also invite your pants to come down.

9. Hi, my name's (your name). Remember it, you'll be screaming it later tonight!

10. Hey, baby, are you wearing your space underwear tonight? Because your ass is out of this world!

12. Hey, sexy. How would you like to join me in doing some math? Let's add you and me, subtract our clothes, divide your legs, and then multiply.

13. Hi, your outfit looks really cute. But it would look even cuter piled on my bedroom floor.

14. Hi, let me interrupt you for a moment. The word of the day is "legs." Let's go back to my place and spread the word.

15. Hi, do you have a little Irish/German/Spanish/Italian/etc. in you? Do you want some?

16. Want to come see my hard drive? I promise it isn't 3.5 inches, and it ain't floppy.

17. I'm an organ donor, and I have an organ you might need.

18. Gorgeous hair. But it'd be even better brushing against my thighs.

19. Wanna play carnival? That's where you sit on my face and I try to guess your weight.

20. If I could rewrite the alphabet, I would put you and I together.

21. There must be something wrong with my eyes—I can't take them off you.

22. Do you have a map? I just keep on getting lost in your eyes.

23. I looked up the word "beautiful" in the thesaurus today, and your name was included.

24. Excuse me, can you give me directions to your heart?

25. Pardon me, but what pickup line works best with you?

26. Excuse me, do you have a quarter I can borrow? I told my mother that I would call her when I fell in love with the girl of my dreams!

27. This is your lucky day, because I just happen to be single.

28. Hi, the voices in my head told me to come over and talk to you.

29. I lost my phone number. Can I borrow yours?

30. Congratulations! You've been voted "Most Beautiful Girl in This Room," and the grand prize is a night with me!

31. Are you religious? Because I'm the answer to your prayers.

32. Are your legs tired? Because you've been running through my mind all day.

33. Is your dad a baker? Because you sure have got great buns.

34. Was your father an alien? Because there's nothing else like you on earth!

35. Did heaven lose a couple of angels? 'Cause I can see them bouncing around in your shirt!

*All right, ladies, any girl who doesn't want to fuck
can leave right now.*

—Babe Ruth upon entering a party

---◆---

Vibrators: The 16 Different Types That Will Shock and Rock Your World

Ah, vibrators. These items can cause erotic magic or scare the prude within. There are many different styles and types of vibrators—so many, in fact, that we couldn't discuss them all in one book. The most popular types are listed with brand names when available. Some are designed for anal stimulation, some to reach the G-spot. Some are meant for the penis and some for the depths of the vagina. There is much information for you, so read on.

1. Wand Vibrators

Wand vibrators are long and slim in shape. They are around one foot in length and have a softball-sized head on the end. They usually vibrate from an electric motor and go at low or high speed. Variations include size, angle, weight, and the size of the head. The most common brands include Wahl, Hitachi, Sunbeam, and Panasonic.

2. Swedish Massager

Remember going to the barber as a kid and the odd device he would use to run over your scalp? Well, if you do then you have a good idea what the Swedish massager looks like. If not, imagine a black box with straps on it that vibrates and is held in the hand. Some men use these devices to stimulate their penis. They can also be used to stimulate the vagina and as a foreplay tool.

3. Battery Vibrators

There are tons of different types of battery-operated vibrators. They tend to be less powerful than electric vibrators, and smaller. Battery vibrators are popular; they are portable and affordable.

4. Egg-shaped Vibrators

These battery powered vibrators look just like a real egg, except they are smaller and made of plastic. They are designed to fit nicely inside the vagina. Some people use them to stimulate the clitoris. Some women wear them inside their underwear.

5. Coil-operated Vibrators

These types of vibrators look like a hairbrush or an electric mixing machine. They are usually around seven inches long and have a long handle. They come with four or five attachments that fit over a metal stub. They are called coil-operated because there is a coil inside that causes the thing to vibrate. Coil-operated vibrators were the first type of vibrator to be available to the general public.

6. Double-headed Vibrators

Similar to the wand vibrators, double headed vibrators offer two ball heads, a few inches apart. This form of vibrator is not very popular and can be difficult to find. They are designed so that users can experience both anal and genital stimulation at once. They have also been used by men who place their penis between the two vibrating balls and also by couples who each claim one of the vibrating balls.

7. Eroscillator Vibrators

This type of vibrator looks like an electric toothbrush. Some report that the vibrations are similar to those emitted from a coil vibrator. Eroscillators are expensive, usually around three times more expensive than the coil vibrator. The head vibrates 360 times per minute.

8. Cylindrical Vibrators

This is the most popular type of vibrator. Most look like a penis, while others are straight and smooth. Some are flexible, and some try to duplicate a penis including veins and color. They are usually made of plastic. They average in size from four inches to eight and most come with attachments.

9. G-spot Vibrators

These type of vibrators are designed to stimulate the G-spot. They have a particular curve and angle that vibrates against the G-spot for added enjoyment. They are similar to cylindrical vibrators.

10. No-hand Vibrators

This class of vibrators is designed to be worn on the leg or waist and to stimulate the clitoris. It was designed to stimulate a woman during intercourse.

11. Vibrating Strap On

This type of vibrator can be strapped onto the leg so that the person wearing it can penetrate his/her partner. Some women penetrate men with such devices. Women also use these devices to penetrate other women. Many people prefer to use strap-on dildos rather than vibrators.

12. Vibrating Sleeve

This device is used by men as a masturbation device. The penis is inserted into the plastic sleeve. There are some that resemble a pair of lips, others look like a vagina, and some are attached to penis pumps.

13. Double Dong

This type of vibrator is designed so that two women can enjoy stimulating each other simultaneously. Other people enjoy using the double-dong to enable anus/anus or anus/vagina stimulation.

14. Anal Vibrator

These are sometimes called "butt plugs" and are quite popular among both women and men. These can be used both for masturbation as well as during sex with a partner. They come in a variety of sizes and colors. One variation is the anal wand. This device is a finger-width bendable device designed to penetrate the anus. (It is important that toys used in the anus be covered with a condom when used.)

15. Nipple-clamp Vibrators

These unorthodox vibrators are used for nipple stimulation. They are attached to the nipples and include adjustable clamps to increase and decrease pressure. They vibrate for added stimulation.

16. Vibrating Cock Ring

This device is a standard cock ring, but has a vibrating egg attached so that the testes are stimulated when the vibrator is turned on. The device is very popular among men.

To read the newspapers and magazines, you would think we were almost worshiping the female bosom.

—Billy Graham

———◆———

Sex Outside: 14 Places You Can Try Today

Warm weather opens up new adventures for even the tamest mind. Most of us will or already have thrown caution to the wind and decided to go for it. We know that the adrenaline-filled thrill and fear of being caught while going at it is all part of outdoor sex. Here is a partial list of places for you to explore; add your own outdoor places of choice to this list and then contact us with your outdoor sexual results.

1. On top of the tallest building in your town. Sneak up in the middle of the night, bring a blanket, and have a romantic night under the stars.

2. Crank up the Grateful Dead and have sex in nature as if it were a drug-induced high. In the process merge with your beloved as if it were the ultimate in spiritual attainment. If there is no natural area near you, sneak into the public gardens for a romp in the azalea bushes.

3. The playground of any park or school yard is a perfect spot for "adult play." Get on the swings and *really* fly. The best device for pleasure is the monkey bars. Check out the monkey business you can get into, in any contorted position. It will be enough to have both of you screaming to the gods for more.

4. The sports fans can go to the bleachers of any football or baseball field and pretend the entire place is watching every gyrating movement. Another option is to go to a ball game and do it under a blanket as everyone else screams and cheers for their favorite player to "score."

5. Parachute naked and somehow end up wrapped up in a frenzy. Strap yourselves together and just let the ride take you quickly down while taking your breath away.

6. For the lazy ones out there, just walk out your damn back door, lie on the ground with a sleeping bag, and go at it.

7. Seek a dark and contemplative cave. Deep in the womb of the earth, you can enter the passion-filled depths under stalagmite and stalactite.

8. Sand on your butt is not so bad when you are getting it on amongst lovers on the beach. Your pubic hair, neck, and

chest covered, and sand castles inspiring summer love on the beach.

9. As the sky is filled with fireworks exploding in colorful streams into the night, you, too, can be exploding in ecstasy. Yes, spend the fourth of July with your sex partner under a blanket at the fireworks show near you.

10. The waves of passion crashing and the moans of your lust sounding like a thousand whales longing to come home—yes, let the water carry you into the depths of sensual lust again. Go out on a boat; specifically, a powerboat at dusk, a canoe in the middle of nowhere, or a raft down a lazy river. Watch out for mosquitoes on private parts; otherwise it will be heavenly.

11. Speaking of wetness and water . . . every outdoor sex freak must have sex in a pool, lake, ocean, or hot tub at least once in his/her sinful career. Jump in and don't worry about the lube.

12. If you really are *true* exhibitionists, climb out on a balcony somewhere you know people can watch and proceed to seduce each other into a fit of naked passion that will carry even the most lame voyeurs into their own private fantasy worlds. Watch out for short guys with video cameras and old ladies with binoculars.

13. The daredevils love to go to the airport and lie down on one end of the runway and shudder under the lights and sounds of planes in flight coming and going into the wide-open sky. Watch out for men in blaze-orange suits; they may want to "direct" you.

14. Your last freaky-deaky adventure can be accomplished by sneaking underneath a dirty and highly trafficked bridge. Have sex under a bridge, amidst the dangers of scumbags and teenagers doing drugs. In the grime of it all, the raw power of sex can emmerge into a dark vampiric passion that even Marilyn Manson would be scared to experience.

*The total exposure of the human body is
undignified as well as an error of taste.*

—Adolf Hitler

———◆———

15 Essential Items for an S/M
Starter Kit

Are you ready to start experimenting with S/M? If so, you better
be prepared. One of the first things you better do is talk to your
partner about what specifically are his/her limits, and then work
within them. Communication is crucial when starting to experiment with S/M or any other form of sexuality.

After you've set up the guidelines and ground rules, you
should then reach into your bag of sex tricks for many of the popular sex devices and toys used in common S/M scenes. Here is an
abbreviated list of some items you may want to purchase and use in
the bedroom.

1. Clothespins

2. Handcuffs

3. Ice

4. Blindfold

5. Belt

6. Flogger

7. Lube

8. Condoms

9. Candles

10. Dog collar

11. Chains

12. Whip

13. Nipple clamps

14. Dildo/butt plug

15. Anal balls

*S&M is deliberate, premeditated,
erotic blasphemy. It is a form of sexual
extremism and sexual dissent.*

—Pat Califia

———◆———

13 Household Items That Can Be Used as Sex Toys

In the mind of even the most sexually tame individual runs the gamut of desires. And in moments of boredom individuals, both kinky and tame, wonder what could enhance sex. We've found items you probably have available to you tonight for your own explorations.

1. Silk ties/scarves

The slippery sensation of ties and scarves can evoke your imagination when they are tied against the velvet skin of your beloved. These items are useful for any blindfolding and bondage experiments. Soft enough so as not to damage skin, yet firm enough to play doctor.

2. Jello®

Jello® is fun and legal. When sprinkled over hard nipples, inner thighs, or pulsating genitalia, miracles and a sticky mess can ensue. Cold and wiggly gelatin can be spread over your lover's chest and slowly ground into his/her stomach as you rub your bodies into a passionate fever. Besides, the raspberry and lime flavors will inevitably evoke the sexual animal within. Throw out the Viagra; Jello® is new the king!

3. Phone

No more messy 900 numbers or expensive phone sex bills—you can now turn your bedroom into a phone-sex palace. For lovers who will not talk about their fantasies, bring two phones into the bedroom and plead with them to pretend you are a phone-sex operator and they are calling in to share their most intimate secrets. Exchange hot words between the sheets.

4. Warm sponge/loofa/vegetable scrubber

Your well-worn and horrifically torn sponge or vegetable cleaner won't save you, but you can use a new unsoiled instrument to first tease the feet and later taunt the genitals of your mate. Abuse your louffa the same way.

5. Spatula

(Don't ask, don't tell.)

6. Paintbrushes

A soft paintbrush can provoke more than mere passion. Go immediately to the hardware store for large and vast selection of these pleasure tools.

7. Ice cubes

For the more sexually demented, ice and other frozen items will bring a shiver and a shock to your honeys. Blindfold them first, and then watch them squirm as you graze their navel, feet, or more provocative areas. Or, place the ice in your mouth and trace lines and circles on various body parts. A truly chilling experience. (Warning: Ice can be dangerous and can burn an individual if left in one spot too long.)

8. Fur

Another sensual delight—rub a furry item (preferably already dead), all over your lover. Focus on the back and buttocks area and then move into the chest, the neck, the feet, and finally . . . the pelvis. In a pinch you can also use anything silky or made with satin.

9. "Sometimes a Cigar Is Just a Cigar."—Freud

For those of you with presidential hopes, reach into the humidor and grab a couple of cigars à la Lewinsky. They seemed to both get off on the action, why wouldn't you?

10. Isopropyl alcohol and cooking oil

Are you ready for weird? Rub either of these substances on body parts for a new sensation. The alcohol will produce a cooling effect, while cooking oil will be warming. Keep both substances away from the eyes and mouth and genitals, however; they could be dangerous.

11. Food

Is your sexual appetite huge? Do you desire the manna of the gods? Maple and chocolate syrup, cucumbers, various fruit, honey, and whipped cream will get anyone in the mood and satisfy your appetite. Use your imagination for interesting scenes you can create for the bedroom, couch, or anywhere else you so desire.

12. Sex-related books, magazines, and videos

Reach into your sock drawer and pull out the latest adult magazine or video to play for your honey. While the prudish will find this a turnoff, it will be an excuse to talk about sex, and your lover will probably agree to make love if only to get you to turn off the video or put the porn magazine away.

13. The shower

For years women have been reporting that they find the strong jets of the shower head produce the strongest orgasms available. So why not utilize this time-tested tip to enhance your own sex life?

Sex is emotion in motion.

—Mae West

───────◆───────

286

6 Love Charms

Charms are usually in the form of bags—talisman bags, medicine bags, ritual bags, and so on, depending on the tradition. These bags are filled with herbs, roots, powders, stones, pieces of cloth, feathers, bones, symbols, hair, and so on. The bag itself is considered a magical object and used in rituals.

1. One love charm used by American voodoo practitioners is called John the Conqueror Root. This root is dried with a spike growing out of it. The spike is an obvious phallic symbol. As a charm, the root is carried in a leather or red cloth bag as a lucky love piece.

2. A Native American love charm is a red and black bag filled with the following herbs: orris root, linden flower, patchouli, violet flower, vervain, rose buds, orange blossoms, and couch grass.

3. An English charm was made by young women to get a man. In one ritual women picked yarrow flowers and placed them in a flannel bag. A woman would then place the bag under her bed before she fell asleep at night. The charm was said to make a wonderful man fall in love with her.

4. Sprinkling powders are another form of love charms. They have been used for ages in love rituals, and call upon spirit powers to aid the seeker in gathering their powers to create the results they desire. Typically, love powders are used in bags that are worn around the neck or are sprinkled around one's home and clothing.

5. Love drawing powder can be used to attract a mate. It is best to chant the name of the person you desire while you mix the powder. Here's the recipe:

1 oz. powdered sandlewood

1/4 tsp. cinnamon

1 tsp. sweet basil

1 tsp. myrtle

1/2 dram frankincense oil

1/2 dram spikenard oil

1 dram red rose oil

4 oz. talc

6. Magic lamps have been used for centuries to help attract spiritual power. They are fueled with castor oil, kerosene, and olive oil. The lamps work in conjunction with prayer.

7. To make a love lamp, start with a fuel that contains equal parts of kerosene, olive oil, and castor. Next add one bottle of love oil, and five-finger grass. Then use a prayer directed toward Saint Anne.

*No man shall marry until he has studied
anatomy and dissected at least one woman.*

—Honore de Balzac (1829)

Sexy Holiday Gifts for Your Lover

If you are like us and hate the holiday season, dread the endless hours of Christmas music, and begin early in November hating the color red, read on. There is one reason to enjoy the holidays: A hidden opportunity to have more sex, of course! For your use and enjoyment, we have selected the hottest gifts available for your sensual pleasure.

Happy Holidays,
Louis and Copeland

1. For the last-minute supper, I mean shopper, there is still hope. The heart's-desire gift basket includes perfume, an easy listening CD, thong, and heart-shaped pillow. (Bright Ideas (888) LUV-4332)

2. Edible Undies will entice the most hungry lovers. Enjoy an edible bra or underwear. Choose from banana, chocolate, mint, and pina-colada flavors. These along with the Mr. Penis Ice Mold are now available. (www.grannny wouldnt.com.

3. Is your lover a twisted sister? Order a sexy vagina or butt-plug soap on a rope. (800-779-3347)

4. Panting for panties? Join the Panty of the Month Club, featuring a designer piece each month, perfumed and gift wrapped. (www.panties.com).

5. Intellectual? *Food as Foreplay* book, $14.95 (800-247-6553)

6. The snow is gently falling outside, and Santa is armed and ready to unveil his new Glow in the Dark Condoms. (Call El Dorado, 800-525-0848)

7. The chestnuts are roasting on an open fire, followed by sweets from the Naughty Baker (608-250-5220). Purchase penis-shaped cakes, breast brownies, and love candy.

8. Celebrate good times—order Remote Control Panties. These leather-harness panties with vibrating bullet inside are designed for a woman, but are strong enough for a man.

Use the long-range remote to make your lover blush any-where, anytime. (Call 1-800-7-SWEDISH to order.)

9. Prepare to take your snow bunny on a love cruise. First Fantasy cruises (805-290-8542) offer four- and seven-day adventures featuring training from romance specialist Shauna Hoffman. These events include fine lingerie, theme wear, tango for lovers, romantic recipes, and more.

10. Stocking stuffer alert! Fill his or her stocking with incense, massage oil, cock rings, pussy lip gloss, lube, vibrating toys, anal beads, and other explicit delights. (http://www.blow-fish.com)

11. The swing: Get out the electric drill and prepare your ceiling for the ultimate weightless sex experience. (888-372-8BUNGEE)

*Love is two minutes fifty-two seconds
of squishing sounds.*

—Johnny Rotten